PHYSIOLOGICAL CHEMISTRY

A Series Prepared under the General Editorship of

Edward J. Masoro, Ph.D.

I PHYSIOLOGICAL CHEMISTRY OF LIPIDS IN MAMMALS

II PHYSIOLOGICAL CHEMISTRY OF PROTEINS AND NUCLEIC ACIDS IN MAMMALS

III ENERGY TRANSFORMATIONS IN MAMMALS: Regulatory Mechanisms

IV ACID-BASE REGULATION: Its Physiology and Pathophysiology

V REGULATION OF AMINO ACID METABOLISM IN MAMMALS

In preparation

PHYSIOLOGICAL CHEMISTRY OF CARBOHYDRATES IN MAMMALS

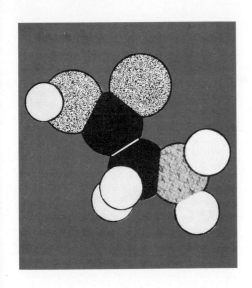

REGULATION OF AMINO ACID METABOLISM IN MAMMALS

Bernard Schepartz, Ph.D.

Professor of Biochemistry,
Jefferson Medical College of
Thomas Jefferson University

1973

W. B. Saunders Company

Philadelphia • London • Toronto

W. B. Saunders Company: West Washington Square
Philadelphia, Pa.   19105

12 Dyott Street
London, WCIA   1DB

833 Oxford Street
Toronto 18, Ontario

Regulation of Amino Acid Metabolism in Mammals   ISBN 0-7216-7955-2

Print No.   9   8   7   6   5   4   3   2   1

Dedication

TO MY WIFE

Who after suffering through four editions of a textbook, and despite my promise of "nevermore," had to endure yet another literary intrusion into our family life.

EDITOR'S FOREWORD

The past three decades or so have seen biochemistry emerge as possibly the most vigorous of the biological sciences. This, in turn, has led to a level of autonomy that has cut the cord linking biochemistry with its historically most important parent, mammalian physiology. For investigators in the fields of both biochemistry and physiology, this vitality has been most useful. But because of the arbitrary separation of these two disciplines in most teaching programs and all textbooks, the vast majority of students do not see the intimate relationships between them. Consequently, the medical student and the beginning graduate student as well as the recently trained physician find it difficult, if not impossible, to utilize the principles of biochemistry as they apply to the physiological and pathological events they observe in man and other mammals.

Therefore, this series is designed not only to introduce the student to the fundamentals of biochemistry but also to show the student how these biochemical principles apply to various areas of mammalian physiology and pathology. It will consist of six monographs: (1) Physiological Chemistry of Lipids in Mammals; (2) Physiological Chemistry of Proteins and Nucleic Acids in Mammals; (3) Energy Transformations in Mammals; (4) Acid-Base Regulation: Its Physiology and Pathophysiology; (5) Regulation of Amino Acid Metabolism in Mammals, the volume herewith presented; and (6) Physiological Chemistry of Carbohydrates in Mammals.

The series can be profitably used by undergraduate medical students. Recent medical graduates and physicians involved in areas of medicine related to metabolism should find that the series enables them to understand the theoretical basis for many of the problems they face in their daily work. Finally, the series should provide students in all areas of mammalian biology with a source of information on the biochemistry of the mammal that is not otherwise currently available in textbook form.

EDWARD J. MASORO

PREFACE

For some years it has appeared to me that the major emphasis of investigators in the field of mammalian metabolism has turned from the search for new metabolic pathways to (1) the regulation and integration of the known metabolic routes into the physiology of the cell and whole organism and to (2) the description of metabolic reactions on the molecular or even electronic level. Whereas there is no shortage of papers, reviews, or monographs along the second route, I have felt for some time that the medical and graduate students in the biomedical sciences had few sources representing the former approach, particularly in my own field of interest, the amino acids.

By a happy coincidence, my feelings along these lines developed at about the time that there began to appear the series of monographs, *Physiological Chemistry*, under Dr. Masoro's editorship and written from the same general point of view. A second coincidence provided the time which made this monograph possible: a sabbatical leave and the loss of financial support for my research.

The subject matter of portions of this monograph has been presented several times over the past few years in the course, Biochemistry 502, Special Topics in Intermediary Metabolism, in the College of Graduate Studies, Thomas Jefferson University.

It is assumed that the reader of this monograph has previously been exposed to an introductory course in animal biochemistry. The work is intended primarily for the use of medical students, graduate students, and workers in the biomedical area who are not specialists in the field of amino acid metabolism (although even those who are may find it a useful review of the current state of the art). Hence, it has seemed most practical to rely chiefly on a bibliography of reviews and monographs, with citations to original articles only when references of the former type are lacking or unsatisfactory.

The term induction is used in an operational sense (cf. Greengard, O.: The quantitative regulation of specific proteins in animal tissues; words and facts. Enzym. Biol. Clin. *8*:81–96, 1967) to mean any increase in the amount or concentration (weight of enzyme per unit weight of tissue) of an enzyme, whether this is due to an increase in the absolute rate of synthesis, a decrease in the rate of degradation, or a combination of the two. Repression is defined in converse fashion. Hence, these terms reflect changes in the *number* of enzyme molecules present in the system. Activation and inhibition are used to indicate an increase and decrease, respectively, in the specific activity of an enzyme *without* a change in concentration, i.e., an alteration in the catalytic properties of those enzyme molecules already present.

Rigorous proof of the mechanism underlying an observed alteration in the activity of an enzyme frequently is not available. Since activation and inhibition appear to be relatively rare in animal tissues, it has been convenient (for purposes of linguistic simplification) to ascribe most changes in apparent enzyme activity, particularly those following hormonal or dietary treatment, to induction and repression, in the absence of evidence to the contrary.

Concerning my choice of content, I confess freely that, after being constrained to defer to the wishes of potential users of four editions of a textbook of biochemistry, I have indulged to the fullest in in the privilege of the monograph writer: I have included that which I found interesting and excluded that which I did not.

B. SCHEPARTZ

CONTENTS

ABBREVIATIONS AND SYMBOLS USED IN FIGURES AND TABLES xiii

CHAPTER 1
INTRODUCTION TO METABOLIC REGULATION 1

CHAPTER 2
OVERALL AMINO ACID METABOLISM 19

CHAPTER 3
AMINO ACID TRANSPORT 33

CHAPTER 4
DEAMINATION, GLUCONEOGENESIS, AND RELATED PATHWAYS.
PART 1: DEAMINATION AND CARBON METABOLISM........................... 51

CHAPTER 5
DEAMINATION, GLUCONEOGENESIS, AND RELATED PATHWAYS.
PART 2: DISPOSAL OF NITROGEN 120

CHAPTER 6
NON-ERGOGENIC PATHWAYS OF AMINO ACID METABOLISM: SELECTED
EXAMPLES 136

INDEX 191

ABBREVIATIONS AND SYMBOLS USED IN FIGURES AND TABLES

Since this monograph is restricted in its coverage to the mammalian organism, the usual prefix, L-, has been omitted from amino acids. In the interest of further typographic simplification, Greek letter prefixes also are omitted where this is not likely to cause confusion.

AA	Amino acid(s)	CHO	Carbohydrate
Ac	Acetyl	CHX	Cycloheximide
AcCoA	Acetyl coenzyme A	CITR	Citrate
AcOAcOH	Acetoacetate	CITRUL	Citrulline
AcOH	Acetate	CoA	Coenzyme A
ACT	Activation	COMT	Catechol O-methyl-transferase
ACT-D	Actinomycin D		
ACTH	Adrenocorticotropic hormone	CORT	Glucocorticoid hormones
Ad	Adenosyl, adenosine	CR	Creatine
ADP	Adenosine diphosphate	CR'N	Creatinine
ADR	Adrenal gland(s)	CR~P	Creatine phosphate
ADREX	Adrenalectomy	CYS	Cysteine
AIB	Aminoisobutyrate	(CYS)$_2$	Cystine
ALA	Alanine	d	Deoxy
ALLYS	Allysine	DAO	Diamine oxidase
AMP	Adenosine monophosphate	DECARB	Decarboxylase
		DEF	Deficiency
cAMP	Cyclic AMP	DH	Dehydrogenase
ANAB	Anabolism, anabolic	DHA	Dihydroxyacetone
ARG	Arginine	DIAB	Diabetes (mellitus)
ASN	Asparagine	DIT	Diiodotyrosine
ASP	Aspartate	DNA	Deoxyribonucleate
ATC	Aspartate transcarbamylase	DOPA	Dihydroxyphenylalanine
ATP	Adenosine triphosphate	DP	Diphosphate
		ENZ	Enzyme
BR-CH	Branched-chain	EPI	Epinephrine
cAMP	Cyclic AMP	ESTRO	Estrogen
CARB~P	Carbamyl phosphate	F	Fructose
CARN	Carnosine	FA	Fatty acid(s)
CARNT	Carnitine	FAA	Fumarylacetoacetate
CATAB	Catabolism, catabolic	FAST	Fasting, starvation

FH$_4$	Tetrahydrofolate
FSH	Follicle-stimulating hormone
FUM	Fumarate
G	Glucose
GABA	(Gamma)-Aminobutyrate
GAL	Galactose
GDH	Glutamate dehydrogenase
GLN	Glutamine
GLU	Glutamate
GLUCAG	Glucagon
GLUCOCORT	Glucocorticoid hormone(s)
GLY	Glycine
GLY'GEN	Glycogen
GLY'OL	Glycerol
GOT	Glutamate-oxaloacetate transaminase
(Alpha)-GP	(Alpha)-Glycerophosphate
G-P	Glucose phosphate(s)
GPT	Glutamate-pyruvate transaminase
GSH	Glutathione (reduced)
GSSG	Oxidized glutathione
GTP	Guanosine triphosphate
GUA	Guanidino
HEPATEX	Hepatectomy
HGA	Homogentisate
HI	High
HIAA	Hydroxyindoleacetate
HIOMT	Hydroxyindole O-methyltransferase
HIS	Histidine
HISTAM	Histamine
HLY	Hydroxylysine
HomoCYS	Homocysteine
HomoSER	Homoserine
HPPA	Hydroxyphenylpyruvate
HPR	Hydroxyproline
HYPOX	Hypophysectomy
ILE	Isoleucine
IM	Imidazole
IN	Indole
IND	Induction
INH	Inhibition
INS	Insulin
IVA	Isovalerate
KA	(Alpha) Keto acid(s)
KG	(Alpha) Ketoglutarate
KGLAM	Ketoglutaramate
KIC	(Alpha) Ketoisocaproate
KID	Kidney(s)
KIV	(Alpha) Ketoisovalerate
KMV	(Alpha) Ketomethylvalerate
LACT	Lactate
LEU	Leucine
LH	Luteinizing hormone
LIV	Liver
LO	Low
LYS	Lysine
MAA	Maleylacetoacetate
MAO	Monoamine oxidase
MELAT	Melatonin
MET	Methionine
METAM	Methiamine
MIT	Monoiodotyrosine
MP	Monophosphate
mRNA	Messenger RNA
MSH	Melanocyte-stimulating hormone
NAD(P)(H)	Nicotinamide adenine dinucleotide (phosphate) (reduced form)
NOREPI	Norepinephrine
OAA	Oxaloacetate
OH-ase	Hydroxylase
ORN	Ornithine
OVARIEX	Ovariectomy
P	Phosphate
PAA	Phenylacetate
PANCREX	Pancreatectomy
PEP	Phosphoenolpyruvate
PHE	Phenylalanine
PLA	Phenyllactate
PNMT	Phenylethanolamine N-methyltransferase
PP	Pyrophosphate
PPA	Phenylpyruvate
PRO	Proline
PROT	Protein
PTER	Pteridine
PTH	Parathyroid hormone
PURO	Puromycin
PUTR	Putrescine
PYR	Pyruvate
R	Ribose
REGEN	Regenerating, regeneration
REP	Repression
RNA	Ribonucleate
rRNA	Ribosomal RNA
SARC	Sarcosine
SER	Serine
SERO	Serotonin
SPER	Spermine
SPERD	Spermidine
STH	Somatotropic (growth) hormone

SUCC	Succinate	TRF	Thyrotropin-releasing factor
T_3	Triiodothyronine		
T_4	Thyroxine	tRNA	Transfer RNA
TA	Transaminase	TRY	Tryptophan
TAU	Taurine	TSH	Thyroid-stimulating hormone
TESTO	Testosterone		
TG	Triglyceride(s)	TYR	Tyrosine
THR	Threonine	UDP	Uridine diphosphate
THYR	Thyroid (gland, hormones)	UTP	Uridine triphosphate
		VAL	Valine
THYREX	Thyroidectomy	XO	Xanthine oxidase
TP	Triphosphate	XS	Excess

$+ + + + + \rightarrow$	Positive influence upon a reaction (ACT or IND)
$- - - - - \rightarrow$	Negative influence upon a reaction (INH or REP)
$\longrightarrow$	Transformation or translocation

1

INTRODUCTION TO METABOLIC REGULATION

CLASSIFICATION OF REGULATORY MECHANISMS

Basic Types of Regulation

Consider the simple catalyzed chemical reaction,

$$A \xrightarrow{\text{ E }} B$$

where A and B are reactant and product, respectively, and E represents an enzyme acting as catalyst. If we define the rate of this reaction as the mass of substrate converted to product per unit time per unit tissue weight, then the rate may be controlled in one or more of the following three ways.

MASS ACTION VARIATIONS. In this most primitive of regulatory mechanisms, the rate of the reaction may be varied by alteration of the concentration of substrate, product (if the reaction is sufficiently reversible so that the concentration of product affects the back-reaction significantly), or any required cofactors which enter into the reaction stoichiometrically.

VARIATION OF SPECIFIC ACTIVITY OF CATALYST. In recent years it has become evident that many enzymes are subject to regulation of their catalytic ability in either or both the positive and negative directions by small molecules which have been called *effectors* or *modulators*. This class of substances includes substrates, products, later metabolites in a path-

1

way, precursors in a pathway, and even metabolites participating in apparently unrelated pathways. In order to standardize nomenclature for later sections of this monograph, the actions of such agents will be termed *activation* and *inhibition* of the enzyme under discussion.

Being virtually instantaneous, the two preceding classes of regulatory mechanisms are sometimes referred to as acute or short-term controls. (Alteration of specific activity of an enzyme under the influence of an effector actually may require a finite amount of time, sometimes seconds to minutes. Enzymes which are slow in this regard have been called *hysteretic*.) Also, since it is commonly believed that these mechanisms, in contrast to the next to be discussed, are capable of very minute alterations, they have been called *fine adjustments* in metabolism.

VARIATION OF CONCENTRATION OF CATALYST.   Although first studied and best established in microorganisms, alterations of the absolute amount of enzyme in a cell is now recognized as one of the major regulatory mechanisms in the animal organism. The instantaneous concentration of an enzyme is the result of the rates of its synthesis and degradation. Although the latter process is of little significance in bacteria, in which an increase in the rate of synthesis is equated with induction, degradative reactions have been shown to be important in regulation of a number of mammalian enzymes. Consequently, in this monograph, an increase in the concentration of an enzyme, for whatever reason, will be defined as *induction* and the corresponding decrease as *repression*.

Regulatory mechanisms involving alterations in the rates of synthesis or degradation of an enzyme consume an appreciable period of time. In the mammal such processes typically have half-times varying from 1 hour to several days. Consequently, such metabolic controls are called chronic or long-term and, in contrast to the preceding classes of mechanisms, are considered *coarse adjustments*.

Biological Levels of Regulation

Since the description of mechanisms of regulation at various biological levels will necessarily involve reference to the component parts of the protein-synthesizing machinery of the cell, it may be appropriate at this point to outline briefly the commonly accepted structures and processes involved.*

NUCLEIC ACIDS AND PROTEIN SYNTHESIS.   The code specifying the amino acid sequence of a given peptide chain is represented in sequences of nucleotides (three nucleotides per amino acid residue) in the deoxyribonucleic acid (DNA) of the genetic apparatus, the genome.

---

*Readers interested in a more detailed description of the process of protein synthesis are referred to the monograph *Physiological Chemistry of Proteins and Nucleic Acids in Mammals* of this series or a textbook of biochemistry.

The DNA molecule consists of two helical polynucleotide strands, held together by hydrogen bonds between complementary bases situated on the two strands (adenine-thymine, guanine-cytosine). Doubling of DNA for mitotic cell division occurs by *replication,* wherein the strands of DNA separate and each serves as a template for synthesis of a complementary strand. The synthesis of a protein begins in a somewhat analogous manner, except that one strand of the DNA serves as template for the synthesis of a complementary strand of messenger ribonucleic acid (mRNA), the complementarity in this case involving a pairing of adenine with uracil (in place of thymine) in the RNA, this synthesis being termed *transcription.* Genomic DNA serves also as template for the synthesis of other species of RNA, such as transfer and ribosomal RNA (tRNA and rRNA, respectively).

Activation of amino acids is the second step in protein synthesis, involving formation of aminoacyl adenylates by reaction with ATP (adenosine triphosphate) and subsequent esterification of the aminoacyl groups with hydroxyl groups of ribose residues in molecules of tRNA. Each tRNA is specific for one amino acid, although most amino acids have several tRNA's of somewhat different structure with which they can combine. In addition to its amino acid–combining site, each tRNA carries a sequence of three nucleotides (an anticodon), the bases of which are complementary to a trinucleotide sequence in mRNA specifying a particular amino acid (a codon).

Without going into details unnecessary for our purpose, the final phase of protein synthesis occurs on the ribosome, where attached mRNA codons attract tRNA anticodons so that the aminoacyl residues which are then linked together have the proper sequence, the genetic information for which was originally specified by the DNA. Actually a number of ribosomes are found combined with each chain of mRNA at any one time, the whole complex being called a *polyribosome* or *polysome.* The conversion of the information embodied in nucleotide sequence to amino acid sequence is termed *translation.*

It is evident from the description above that the process of protein synthesis presents many areas which may be subject to regulatory influences.

LEVELS OF SOPHISTICATION. The most primitive living organisms are the prokaryotes (bacteria and blue-green algae), which are characterized by the absence of a true nucleus and other intracellular organelles such as mitochondria and endoplasmic reticulum. Even in these apparently simple cells, a host of regulatory mechanisms can be found, such as control of transport across the cell membrane and activation, inhibition, induction, and repression of enzymes. Although these organisms contain nuclear regions, no membrane separates the genome from the cytoplasm. As a consequence, transcription and translation may occur in close juxtaposition, and many cytoplasmic regulatory influences may be brought to bear directly upon the DNA, whereas in nucleated cells these influences may be forced to adopt more indirect routes.

Eukaryotes, even of the unicellular variety (e.g., yeasts), present a much more complex picture. Owing to the enclosure of the genome within a nuclear membrane, as well as the presence of mitochondria, endoplasmic reticulum, and other organized intracellular structures, compartmentation of enzymes and metabolic pathways occurs. This makes possible regulation of transport across the limiting membranes of intracellular organelles. In addition, segregation of the genome from the cytoplasm probably results in the development of more mechanisms of induction-repression on the translational level in contrast to the prokaryotes, where this type of regulation appears to be mostly transcriptional.

A major difference in the genomic environment between eukaryotes and prokaryotes is the envelopment of the nuclear DNA of the former by basic proteins (protamines or histones), a characteristic which may have regulatory implications in the higher forms of life, in which a large proportion of the genome is nonfunctional at any given time.

Multicellular eukaryotes, which term includes all of the higher plants and animals, require additional regulatory mechanisms to cope with their greater complexity. Since there is a division of labor among the cells of such organisms, it is necessary for mechanisms to exist which will control differentiation of cells during development, ensuring, for example, that a nerve cell will be provided with the structural and metabolic machinery which will enable it to function as a nerve cell. Multicellularity also produces problems of intercellular communication. Since different types of cells in different locations are performing different tasks, it is essential to the survival of the organism, and to the eventual survival of the species in evolution, that integrative controls exist which can regulate the function of the parts for the good of the whole. These controls are of two types, signals of a chemical (hormonal) or of an electrical (neuronal) nature.

ILLUSTRATION OF REGULATORY MECHANISMS

Figure 1–1 depicts examples of the types of mechanisms enumerated in the preceding sections and, incidentally, illustrates the graphic conventions to be used in the remainder of this monograph to indicate the several kinds of regulatory factors and their sites of action. The following comments on the mechanisms shown in the figure (and on a few omitted for simplification) will proceed, in general, from the simple to the complex.

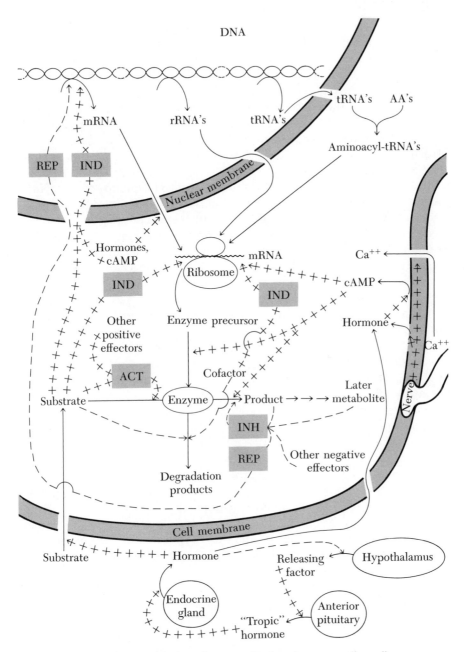

Figure 1–1. Typical regulatory mechanisms in a mammalian cell.

**Mechanisms Involving Constant Concentration of
Enzyme, Nongenomic**

MASS ACTION.   Most enzymes are not present in the cell in limiting concentrations, hence the rate of the reaction catalyzed by each is determined by the rate at which substrate is supplied. (If the reaction is readily reversible, the rate of removal of product by subsequent reactions may be of importance.) An example of this mechanism, on a rather complex level, is the control of the rate of gluconeogenesis in liver by the rate of delivery of amino acids, especially alanine, from peripheral muscle. Of course, this mechanism simply moves the site of actual control to another location: one must determine what alters the rate of supply of substrate in the first place.

Participation of a substrate, and even more frequently a coenzyme, in more than one metabolic pathway can result in regulation by competition, a so-called "bottleneck" effect. The final effect of this competition is exerted via the mass action mechanism. A readily demonstrated *in vitro* example, which some believe to have medical implications in hepatic coma, is the inhibition of function of the Krebs cycle when mitochondria are treated with ammonium salts. Ketoglutarate, a member of the cycle, is withdrawn into another metabolic pathway by being converted, first to glutamate, then to glutamine, by successive reaction with two molecules of ammonia.

STRUCTURAL FACTORS, TRANSPORT.   Compartmentation of the interior of the cell into a soluble phase plus numerous organelles makes possible many regulatory mechanisms of a segregational type. Rates of transport of molecules and ions across the cell membrane and into and out of organelles are frequently regulated and in turn regulate the rates of reactions dependent upon the concentrations of the substances being transported. An example is the facilitation by insulin of amino acid transport into the cells of skeletal muscle.

In quite another structural aspect of regulation, the aggregation of all of the enzymes of a metabolic sequence into a multi-enzyme particle (e.g., the pyruvate dehydrogenase complex) or into the interior of an organelle (Krebs cycle, oxidative chain) not only confers on the system superior kinetics as compared with random collisions in free solution but also allows coordinated regulation of the sequence of reactions as one unit.

MODULATION OF ENZYME ACTIVITY.   An enzyme early in a metabolic sequence often is found to be inhibited by the product of a reaction much later in the sequence. Since the structure of the inhibitor generally bears little or no resemblance to that of the substrate of the inhibited enzyme, it has been concluded that the inhibited site differs from the catalytic site, hence the term *allosteric*. Regulatory mechanisms of this type, whereby the concentration of a metabolite acts as a signal to the machinery producing that metabolite in such a way that an increase in concentration decreases the rate of production, are examples of *negative feedback,* a term borrowed from engineering. For reasons which will be discussed later, the name *end-product inhibition,* which is often applied to these cases, may be a poor choice. *Metabolite inhibition* may be better.

Further investigation has widened the roster of negative effectors or modulators of enzymes to include the immediate product of the inhibited reaction as well as substances apparently having no direct metabolic relation to the enzyme in question.

Positive allosteric effectors also are known, and include compounds occurring earlier in the metabolic sequence than the reaction affected, the substrate of the activated enzyme itself (presumably acting at the allosteric, not the catalytic, site), and again, apparently unrelated substances. It may be noted that unrelated effectors of both the positive and negative types frequently are members of other metabolic pathways, and hence may be playing integrative roles between one route of metabolism and another.

Since allosteric sites are distant from and not covalently connected with catalytic sites, allosteric effects must be exerted through conformational changes in the protein molecule. Although there would appear to be no intrinsic obstacle to such alterations occurring within a single peptide chain, the most thoroughly studied allosteric proteins up to this time have proved to be composed of subunit peptide chains, with the allosterism involving some alteration in the steric relationship among the subunits, accompanied by alterations within the subunits.

Frequently it is found that binding of one molecule of effector by an allosteric protein facilitates the binding of additional molecules. This is called a cooperative effect.

The phenomenon of allosterism is not confined to enzymes. Indeed, the most familiar example is hemoglobin, the binding of oxygen causing allosteric changes among and within the four subunits as well as exhibiting the property of cooperativity.

Mechanisms Involving Variable Concentration of Enzyme, Genomic

Initially the terms induction and repression were applied exclusively to these genomic mechanisms, since, in the growing bacterium where they were being studied, no significant amount of degradation took place. With the wider definition used in this monograph, these mechanisms are perhaps better designated as *nuclear, genomic,* or *transcriptional* induction and repression.

The bacterial genetic machinery required for turning out the specifications of a given inducible or repressible enzyme is believed to consist of (a) the sequence of nucleotides necessary to code for the sequence of amino acids in the final peptide chain, the so-called *structural gene*, (b) a switching unit which turns on or off the process of transcription of the structural gene, the *operator*, and (c) a *regulator gene* which, through a protein intermediary, and in the absence of other influences, keeps the switch in the "normally off" or "normally on" position. The complex of operator plus structural gene (or genes, since transcription of mRNA for several peptide chains may be controlled by one operator) is called an *operon*.

In the most thoroughly studied system, the inducible *lac* operon of *Escherichia coli,* the regulator gene produces a repressor protein, which prevents the operator from switching on the transcription of structural genes. Positive effectors, inducers, combine with the repressor and modify it in such a way (believed to be allosteric) that it can no longer block the operator. In similarly constructed repressible systems, the repressor does not function until modified by co-repressors, which are negative effectors. It will be noted that, in this negative type of regulatory system, induction actually amounts to inhibition of a repression.

Negative control systems are not universal, even among bacteria. Certain operons exist which appear to have switching mechanisms operating in the "normally on" mode; hence the product of their regulator genes must be an inducer protein, and the systems will have properties exactly opposite to those described above.

Whichever mechanism happens to apply to a given inducible or repressible enzyme, it is obvious that the rate of synthesis of that enzyme, being dependent upon the presence of the appropriate mRNA, will in turn be dependent upon the presence or absence of effectors or modulators, which can thus alter the concentration of enzyme to adapt the cell to a particular set of metabolic circumstances.

How much of this scheme can be carried over from bacteria to the mammal is problematic at this time. On the one hand, it would be very unlikely for most of the properties of so fundamental a unit as the genome not to be found, albeit somewhat altered, in all forms of life. On the other, there is no doubt that the basic conditions of life are very different for the growing bacterium and for the multicellular eukaryote. It will be assumed in this monograph that the mammalian cell possesses something akin to an operon system, functioning in transcriptional induction and repression, but that, in the course of evolutionary change, new types of post-transcriptional control have been developed. For example, with the existence of a nuclear membrane, it becomes possible to control the rate of efflux of mRNA to the cytoplasm. In addition, translational controls exist, some of which may have their origins in nuclear events. Variation in the amounts of rRNA or tRNA made or exported may be considered in this category.

Certain cases of induction and repression in bacteria involve multiple enzymes, often the entire group of enzymes catalyzing consecutive steps in a metabolic sequence. This phenomenon, called coordinate induction or repression in bacteria, may have its counterpart in higher forms of life. Thus, all the enzymes of the ornithine cycle in mammalian liver are induced by increasing the protein content of the diet.

Enzyme synthesis in bacteria sometimes can be repressed by the presence of glucose. This glucose effect is thought to be mediated by the increased concentrations of the many catabolites of glucose, and the term *catabolite repression* has been applied. There is no generally accepted explanation of the analogous effect of administration of glucose to animals which results in the repression of the catabolism of several gluconeogenic amino acids. In the animal organism more complex mechanisms may be involved, including the participation of hormones and cAMP.

The inhibitor, actinomycin D, which interferes with the synthesis of RNA on a DNA template, often is used to pinpoint the site of a given regulatory influence as transcriptional, specifically in regard to the synthesis of mRNA. Although this interpretation is perfectly valid in many cases (supported by additional evidence), the situation is not always unambiguous. At the lowest concentrations, actinomycin appears to inhibit the synthesis of rRNA. Concentrations which are inhibitory to the synthesis of mRNA are at the toxic, even lethal, level, which raises the possibility of unanticipated and unwanted side effects. An additional complication in the use of this inhibitor is its ability, in certain systems, to block degradative reactions, presumably at some post-translational site.

In addition to repressors (or co-repressors) and inducers (or co-inducers) such as substrates and their precursors or analogs and products and their analogs, some hormones are believed to function at the transcriptional site. An example is the induction of tyrosine transaminase in liver by adrenal glucocorticoid hormones, an effect which is inhibited by actinomycin and for which there is some evidence, although indirect, of the expected acceleration in synthesis of mRNA. It should be mentioned also at this point that some hormones may act at the nuclear level by controlling the efflux of specific mRNA's from the nucleus, whereas others eventually have an effect at the genomic site by way of an intermediary, such as cAMP.

Mechanisms Involving Variable Concentration of Enzyme, Nongenomic

REGULATION OF NUMBER OF FUNCTIONAL CELLS. This mechanism has been suggested for the regulation of the rate of synthesis of albumin and other plasma proteins by the liver, particularly in response to varying influx of amino acids. The results of the experiments, which were based on fluorescent antibody techniques, are subject to a number of interpretations; hence, this otherwise attractive regulatory mechanism cannot be regarded as established as yet.

REGULATION AT THE tRNA LEVEL. Nothing is known concerning

factors controlling nuclear production of the various species of tRNA, their export to the cytoplasm, or their stability or function in the cytoplasm. However, histidine biosynthesis in a bacterial system is repressed by histidyl-rRNA, suggesting the possibility in animal cells that the concentrations of aminoacyl-tRNA's may have some regulatory significance, in this case on the translational level.

REGULATION AT THE RIBOSOMAL LEVEL.   Mammalian mRNA's generally have longer lives than those of bacteria and differ greatly among themselves as well in this respect. Whether the stability of a given mRNA may be controlled is not known.

The aggregation of individual ribosomes with mRNA to form polysomes in the liver is greatly influenced by the supply of free amino acids, particularly tryptophan (present in limiting concentration in liver), thus providing a mechanism for accelerating hepatic protein synthesis at a time when the raw materials are plentiful, i.e., during digestion and absorption of a protein-containing meal.

Although it is not certain that the supply of ribosomes as such exerts a controlling influence upon the rate of protein synthesis, it may be noted that treatment of an animal with glucocorticoids, in addition to whatever specific effects may be exerted on certain mRNA's, results in a greatly enhanced rate of synthesis of hepatic rRNA. It is also possible that the specific protein synthesizing capacity of ribosomes is under endocrine control. Ribosomes from muscle of diabetic animals exhibit a decreased capability of incorporating amino acids into protein, a defect which can be prevented by pre-treatment of the animals with insulin.

In contrast to the action of actinomycin discussed earlier, the inhibitors puromycin and cycloheximide function at the ribosomal site. Any regulatory mechanism blocked by these substances is assumed to operate at the translational level.

Examples are known of post-transcriptional induction at either the translational or post-translational level by substrates, coenzymes and prosthetic groups, and hormones. It has been theorized that a substrate or cofactor, by combination with the nascent peptide chain, may facilitate the folding of the latter into its functional conformation, thus removing it from the polysome more rapidly, or in some other way preventing it from "clogging" the protein-manufacturing machinery.

REGULATION OF RATE OF DEGRADATION.   Induction, as defined in this monograph, may result from either a differential increase in the rate of synthesis of a protein, a differential decrease in its rate of degradation, or a combination of the two. Examples of all three modes of induction are known.

The theory that combination of an enzyme (or apoenzyme) with its substrate or coenzyme (or prosthetic group) alters the conformation of the protein so as to protect it from whatever degradative mechanisms may exist has a rather long history, although supportive evidence has only recently become available. A well-documented example is the induction of tryptophan pyrrolase by tryptophan, which has been shown conclusively to be due entirely to stabilization of the enzyme against degradation.

In contrast to the wealth of detailed information on the mechanism of protein synthesis, little is known concerning the pathway of intracellular degradation. Although assumed to be proteolytic, possibly catalyzed by the *cathepsins* (lysosomal proteinases), the process has been reported to require energy, being inhibited by anaerobiosis or "uncoupling" agents. Recent investigations have indicated that the energetic requirement relates to some structural component of the system, not to the purely catalytic factors. In connection with the possible participation of lysosomes, it is of interest that glucocorticoids, which generally favor protein catabolism (with the exception of certain inductive actions on specific enzymes), stabilize the lysosomal membranes.

REGULATION OF SECRETION. It is believed by some that proteins which are destined for export from the cell are synthesized on polysomes attached to membranes of the endoplasmic reticulum, in contrast to those intended for intracellular use, which are synthesized on unattached polysomes. Whatever the case, the former group of proteins travels via the channels of the endoplasmic reticulum to the Golgi apparatus for secretion. In those proteins which require carbohydrate prosthetic groups (glycoproteins), the carbohydrate is attached sequentially to the peptide chain as it passes from the ribosomes through the endoplasmic reticulum and cell membrane. Many secretable proteins, particularly if they are highly biologically active molecules, such as hormones or enzymes, are packaged and kept in reserve in storage granules, waiting for the regulatory stimulus which releases them through the cell membrane.

Although in many cases it is difficult to disentangle regulatory influences which affect the synthesis of a protein from those which stimulate its secretion, a clear-cut example of the latter is the insulin-releasing effect of glucose and glucagon on the beta cells of the pancreas, in both cases proceeding via the intermediary, cAMP.

REGULATION BY CHEMICAL MODIFICATION. Some enzymes are catalytically active almost immediately after synthesis, with due allowance for the short time required for folding into their native conformations, aggregation of subunit peptide chains, and attachment of prosthetic groups. Others are activated only by alterations of a chemical nature. These alterations may be regulatory in that they produce an active enzyme *when* and *where* required by the organism.

The best example of the locational type of regulation is provided by the mammalian proteolytic digestive enzymes (pepsin, trypsin, chymotrypsin), which are secreted in the form of inactive zymogens. The inactive zymogens are converted to the active enzymes by cleavage of peptide bonds, under the influence of agents such as acid or other enzymes which are found in the locations where the proteinases are destined to function. Thus, digestion occurs where desired and not where the action could be harmful, such as in the cell of origin.

The biological activities of certain proteins can be altered by addition or removal of small chemical groups, such as methyl, acetyl, and phosphoryl. Phosphorylation appears to be a means of activation of a number of enzymes (e.g., phosphorylase, involved in glycogenolysis), catalyzed by protein kinases, many of which in turn have been shown to be activated by a compound now attracting much interest, cAMP (adenosine $3',5'$-monophosphate).

Formation of cAMP is catalyzed by adenyl cyclase, an enzyme found bound to the cell membrane and the membranes of the endoplasmic reticulum:

$$ATP \longleftrightarrow cAMP + pyrophosphate$$

Since the cyclase of a given tissue is activated by hormones known to act upon that tissue, since the intracellular concentration of cAMP is elevated by the hormonal treatment, and since the actions of the hormones can be mimicked by treating the tissue directly with cAMP, it has been hypothesized that the actions of many hormones proceed via cAMP, a "second messenger."

Degradation of cAMP is catalyzed by a phosphodiesterase, found largely in the soluble phase of the cytoplasm:

$$cAMP + H_2O \longrightarrow 5'\text{-}AMP + phosphate$$

This enzyme is characteristically inhibited by methylxanthines (caffeine, theophylline), which, therefore, potentiate the action of cAMP or any agent producing it. Such potentiation has been used as a clue to the involvement of cAMP in various biological processes.

Calcium ions are in some way related to the function of cAMP. The stimulus to the cell membrane which activates adenyl cyclase also appears to increase the permeability of the membrane to the influx of calcium ions, cAMP liberates calcium ions from intracellular stores, and the presence of calcium ions appears to be essential for many of the final effects of cAMP.

Additional cytoplasmic roles for cAMP which have been suggested include the allosteric activation of enzymes, the chemical modification of enzymes, and, in some unknown fashion, acceleration of the translational process at the ribosome.

As indicated in an earlier section, the inductive action of certain hormones appears to be exerted at the genomic level, but by way of cAMP as intermediary. In this connection it is of interest that cAMP promotes phosphorylation of nuclear histones, those basic proteins which coat the nuclear DNA and probably keep much of its genetic information in the repressed state. It is possible that such phosphorylation is a part of the genomic inductive system.

From the standpoint of comparative biochemistry, it is of interest that cAMP is identical with acrasin, an agent which induces aggregation of cellular slime molds and is also responsible for attracting these molds to certain bacteria. In the latter organisms cAMP has been found to function in inductive processes at both the transcriptional and translational levels.

Miscellaneous Regulatory Mechanisms

ISOZYMES. Isoenzymes or isozymes are structurally different enzymes which catalyze the same reaction. They are involved in metabolic regulation in several ways. For example, one isozymic form of an enzyme may be present in the mitochondria, another in the cytoplasm. The mitochondrial enzyme may be closely related to the oxidative chain or in some other way required to be present in relatively constant concentration, whereas the cytoplasmic enzyme, although catalyzing the same chemical reaction, may be part of another metabolic pathway. As such, the latter enzyme may be amenable to control by way of either induction-repression or activation-inhibition.

Cases are known in which the fetal and adult forms of an enzyme are different. Presumably, the properties of each isozymic variant are adapted to the physiological needs of the organism at each stage of development.

In certain branched metabolic pathways in bacteria an enzyme functioning before the branch-point may occur in several isozymic forms, each sensitive to inhibition or repression (or both) by an end product of one of the branches. As a result the reaction catalyzed, although it may be decreased in overall rate by one end product, is not completely blocked unless there is a surplus of all products. This mechanism is usually supplemented by more specific controls in each pathway after the branch-point.

It has been demonstrated in several instances in which an enzyme exists in the form of multiple isoenzymes, and in which induction of synthesis of the enzyme is under the influence of several regulatory factors, that each isoenzyme responds specifically and independently to one of the regulators. It is too early to say whether these observations will lead to a new generalization or law of metabolic regulation, but the situation bears watching.

ENDOCRINE MECHANISMS OF REGULATION. Although hormonal (or more broadly, humoral) mechanisms of regulation arose in evolution for intercellular communication in multicellular organisms, these mechanisms operate by way of the same basic intracellular means found in simpler forms of life. It is doubtful if any hormone exerts its effect by reacting directly with an enzyme. These regulators function rather by altering the permeability of a membrane to a metabolite, by inducing at the nuclear level (probably by allosteric interaction with repressor or inducer proteins), or by way of cAMP, which in turn may function at the nuclear, ribosomal, or post-translational level.

It has been suggested that two general mechanisms exist for hormonal action on the molecular level. The first of these, as demonstrated by the behavior of certain polypeptide hormones (e.g., glucagon) and the catecholamines (e.g., epinephrine), functions at the cell membrane, where it alters the activity of adenyl cyclase. The resultant alteration in the intracellular level of cAMP in turn brings about various consequences which are noted elsewhere. The second general mechanism has been shown to operate most conclusively in the case of the estrogens and progesterone, with some evidence that it is of significance also in the case of other steroid hormones, such as androgens, glucocorticoids, and aldosterone. The steroid hormones appear to enter the cell, where each combines with a specific receptor protein. The complex then enters the nucleus, a process which, in certain cases at least, requires some alteration in the properties of the receptor (allosteric modification by the steroid?). Interaction of the complex with the genome seems to occur, since there is observed an acceleration of the process of transcription (enhanced activity of RNA polymerase). The specificity of the interaction remains to be elucidated.

It is highly probable that additional hormonal mechanisms exist. Certain actions of insulin are not explicable by the cAMP mechanism, for example. In addition, the probable post-transcriptional regulation of tyrosine transaminase and tryptophan pyrrolase (Chapter 4) by glucocorticoids would appear to require considerable supplementation of the second mechanism outlined in the previous paragraph.

It should be noted that the synthesis and secretion of hormones themselves provide examples of regulation, often of the negative feedback type. The stimulus for secretion of certain hormones, for example, begins with the arrival of a humoral or electrical signal at the hypothalamus, from which a hypothalamic releasing factor is sent to the anterior pituitary gland. This gland then secretes (among other things) a "tropic" hormone (e.g., thyrotropic, adrenocorticotropic) which, acting upon the target endocrine gland, stimulates production and/or secretion of the hormone in question. This final product, once in the circulation, often interacts with the hypothalamus to suppress the entire chain of events, hence the cycle becomes self-regulating.

NEURAL REGULATION. As in the case of the preceding group of mechanisms, the intercellular controls operating by way of the nervous system do so by intracellular means. Thus, an arriving nerve impulse has no direct influence upon an enzyme. Instead, the electrical signal is transduced to a chemical signal, such as increased flux of one or more inorganic ions, or release of a neurohormone, the ultimate result being the dispatch of a second messenger such as cAMP to carry out what is recognized as the physiological effect of the neural stimulation. The release of neurohormones themselves may require participation of cAMP.

RHYTHMIC REGULATION. The concentrations of certain substances in blood plasma (amino acids, glucocorticoid hormones) and of certain enzymes in liver (tyrosine transaminase) undergo daily variations in magnitude (diurnal rhythmicity), the period of oscillation being approximately 24 hours (circadian).

Many instances of rhythmic biological phenomena are due to the interaction of two factors, one endogenous and the other exogenous to the organism. The endogenous factor provides the basic drive, which may result in a phenomenon exhibiting periodicity of approximately 1 day, as in the case of tyrosine transaminase. In the instance cited, the endogenous drive is unknown (perhaps residing in the central nervous system), but its effect is to cause rats to eat in rhythmic fashion. The exogenous factor, which may be a periodic food supply, periodic cycles of illumination, etc., entrains the endogenous drive and keeps it in synchrony. Such a factor has been termed a *Zeitgeber*.

DEVELOPMENTAL REGULATION. It is generally accepted that differentiation of multicellular organisms involves programmed, sequential activation of genes. Unfortunately, little is known of the regulatory mechanisms on a molecular level.

Differentiation of an embryonic tissue often is dependent upon exogenous factors, embryonic inducers, which diffuse from an adjacent tissue. Identification of the active substances has been the object of much controversy and is still being vigorously pursued.

Apparently hormones are among the substances which can act as inducers during the fetal stage of mammalian development. Administration of a hormone (e.g., glucagon) to a fetal rat can induce the synthesis of an enzyme (tyrosine transaminase) in the liver before its normal time of appearance. However, inducing agents are each effective only at characteristic stages of development, hence they require a certain competence of the tissues involved. The factors which program this competence are unknown.

Although first causes remain to be discovered, much useful information is being collected on the developmental patterns of enzymes and metabolic pathways. In the *de novo* appearance of enzymes in mammalian liver the enzymes seem to occur in clusters, each group making its debut at a time coinciding with a significant alteration in the physiological state of the animal. In the rat the important developmental stages are (1) late fetal, during which period many endocrine glands become functional; (2) neonatal, at which time the organism must acclimate itself to aerobiosis plus the loss of maternal nutrition; and (3) late suckling or weaning, when a drastic change occurs in the nature of the food intake, along with certain further endocrine developments.

SOME REGULATORY FOLKLORE

It was originally believed, on the basis of insufficient evidence, that inductive mechanisms were characteristic of catabolic pathways and repressive mechanisms were characteristic of anabolic pathways. Aside from the difficulty of classifying metabolic pathways in one category or the other, the accumulated evidence now indicates that the reactions of a metabolic pathway may be under any of many known types of regulation.

Many metabolic pathways contain branch-points, hence the chain of reactions cannot be said to lead exclusively to a specific product unless one begins demarcating reactions after the last bifurcation. The first reaction in this limited series is known as the *committed step,* since the compounds undergoing the reactions from this point on are destined to form only the product in question. It would be physiologically economical for the committed step to be the site of regulatory mechanisms, and indeed, this is frequently the case. Unfortunately, the step designated as committed is sometimes so identified on the basis of already available metabolic maps, assuming that no later bifurcations exist in the series of reactions. On occasion, this assumption has never been tested through the use of isotopes or by any other means.

Reference has been made earlier to the terms end-product inhibition and end-product repression. In this monograph end product has been replaced by metabolite, a change justified by the observation that many (if not most) so-called end products are not, in fact, end products insofar as the organism is concerned. The term is anthropomorphic, unfortunately reflecting the "end" of a man-made pathway, which in the organism is by no means a stopping place. Probably the best example which could be cited is the pathway of biosynthesis of any amino acid, where this extraordinarily biologically reactive metabolite, with many metabolic pathways open to it, is somehow regarded as an end product.

Reactions which are physiologically irreversible (i.e., have large equilibrium constants), since they can function as unidirectional valves in the flow of metabolic materials, would seem to be logical sites for the operation of regulatory mechanisms. This expectation is realized in many instances. However, these observations cannot be raised to the level of a generalization, since the rate of a reaction seems to have more regulatory significance than its equilibrium properties.

In a sequence of chemical reactions the rate of overall conversion of initial reactants to final products is determined by the slowest step, known as the *rate-limiting* reaction. Once a steady state is achieved, and assuming that substrates and cofactors are not in limited supply, then all reactions in the sequence will operate at the same rate, that of the rate-limiting step. As might be anticipated, rate-limiting reactions are frequent targets of regulatory influences, even when they are freely reversible.

It is frequently found that, even when a committed step is regulated, several later steps in the pathway are also regulated. When a metabolite (such as the anthropomorphic end product) exerts negative feedback inhibition or repression upon an earlier reaction, other metabolites in the pathway may do the same. When a rate-limiting reaction is regulated, other reactions in the sequence which are not rate-limiting may also be regulated. Evidently some principle of regulatory redundancy is at work in these cases, which are far from exceptional. Two possible explanations for these observations come to mind:

1. Redundant regulatory mechanisms are vestigial remains of methods of metabolic control which were of importance in the distant evolutionary past and have been carried along because they present no threat to survival. Since certain metabolic pathways probably belong to this vestigial category, there is no *a priori* reason to exclude regulatory mechanisms. However, the large number of cases of redundancy militates against this explanation.

2. Regulatory redundancy is itself an aid to evolutionary survival, since it protects the organism against changes in conditions which may render the primary regulatory mechanism ineffective. This explanation seems the more probable. Taking as an example the control of rate-limiting reactions, it is not unusual for several other reactions in a metabolic sequence to be almost as slow as the slowest. Perturbations in the concentrations of substrates, cofactors, or concentration or activity of other enzymes all may shift the focus of regulation from the primary to a secondary site.

REFERENCES

General Mechanisms of Regulation

Weber, G. (ed.): Advances in Enzyme Regulation. Oxford, Pergamon Press, Ltd, annual volumes beginning with Vol. 1, 1963.

Koshland, D. E., Jr., and Neet, K. E.: The catalytic and regulatory properties of enzymes. Ann. Rev. Biochem. 37:359–410 (1968).

San Pietro, A., Lamborg, M. R., and Kenney, F. T. (eds.): Regulatory Mechanisms for Protein Synthesis in Mammalian Cells. New York, Academic Press, Inc., 1968.

Horecker, B. L., and Stadtman, E. R. (eds.): Current Topics in Cellular Regulation. New York, Academic Press, Inc., serial publication beginning with Vol. 1, 1969.

Litwack, G. (ed.): Biochemical Actions of Hormones. Vol. 1. New York, Academic Press, Inc., 1970. Vol. 2, 1972.

Munro, H. N. (ed.): Mammalian Protein Metabolism. Vol. 4. New York, Academic Press, Inc., 1970.

Schimke, R. T., and Doyle, D.: Control of enzyme levels in animal tissues. Ann. Rev. Biochem. 39:929–976 (1970).

Rechcigl, M., Jr. (ed.): Enzyme Synthesis and Degradation in Mammalian Systems. Baltimore, University Park Press, 1971.

Robison, G. A., Butcher, R. W., and Sutherland, E. W.: Cyclic AMP. New York, Academic Press, Inc., 1971.

Vogel, H. J. (ed.): Metabolic Pathways. Vol. 5. Metabolic Regulation. New York, Academic Press, Inc., 1971.

Kun, E., and Grisolia, S. (eds.): Biochemical Regulatory Mechanisms in Eukaryotic Cells. New York, Wiley-Interscience, 1972.

Pitot, H. C., and Yatvin, M. B.: Interrelationships of mammalian hormones and enzyme levels in vivo. Physiol. Rev. *53*:228–325 (1973).

Schimke, R. T.: Control of enzyme levels in mammalian tissues. Adv. Enz. *37*:135–187 (1973).

Developmental Regulation

Bonner, J.: The Molecular Biology of Development. New York, Oxford University Press, 1965.

Weber, R. (ed.): The Biochemistry of Animal Development. Vol. 1. New York, Academic Press, Inc., 1965. Vol. 2, 1967.

Florkin, M., and Stotz, E. H. (eds.): Comprehensive Biochemistry. Vol. 28. Morphogenesis, Differentiation, and Development. Amsterdam, Elsevier Publishing Company, 1967.

Gross, P. R.: Biochemistry of differentiation. Ann. Rev. Biochem. *37*:631–660 (1968).

Knox, W. E.: Enzyme Patterns in Fetal, Adult, and Neoplastic Tissues. Basel, S. Karger, 1972.

2

OVERALL AMINO ACID METABOLISM

INTRODUCTION

A thorough treatment of amino acid metabolism involves detailed consideration of the metabolic pathways of some 20 compounds, many of which participate in multiple metabolic routes. The sheer number of observations available in this area, however, even when summarized in the form of metabolic flow-diagrams, tends to obscure the large picture. It is essential, therefore, in an overall survey, to differentiate the major processes from the minor.

The average 70-kg man in technologically advanced countries may consume as much as 100 gm of protein per day, containing about 16 gm (more than 1 gm-atom) of amino acid nitrogen. Of this turnover of over 1000 mmoles of amino acids per day, only processes involving 10 per cent or more of this total can reasonably be considered major participants. Such processes include digestion and the internal turnover of protein in the gastrointestinal tract, the anabolic transformation of amino acids into the proteins of plasma and tissues, the catabolism of amino acids to yield energy and waste products (including the intermediate pathway of gluconeogenesis), and the translocation of amino acid nitrogen from one tissue to another. This chapter and those immediately following will concentrate upon these major pathways.

For the purposes of this chapter it may be profitable to delimit the field even further. A perfectly satisfactory and useful picture of the grand design of amino acid metabolism in the mammalian organism can be constructed on the physiological or supramolecular level, considering chiefly the direction of flow of the major processes mentioned above and its regulation by dietary and hormonal factors. Detailed treatment of the mechanism of each regulatory factor on the molecular level, e.g., consideration of whether a given factor operates through an influence upon an active transport system or by activating an enzyme or by causing increased synthesis of an enzyme, will be deferred to subsequent chapters.

Since the mass flow of amino acid nitrogen (as defined above) quantitatively takes place chiefly within and among a restricted number of organs or tissues, it is necessary to describe the role of each of these areas in amino acid metabolism before consideration of their interrelations and the role of regulatory factors.

ROLE OF INDIVIDUAL ORGANS

Gastrointestinal Tract (Fig. 2-1)

Details of the process of digestion of proteins may be found in the monograph, *Physiological Chemistry of Proteins and Nucleic Acids in Mammals,* in this series, or in any standard textbook of biochemistry. It will suffice at this point to state that proteins of the diet are hydrolyzed in the lumen of the gastrointestinal tract, under the influence of proteinases and peptidases originating in the gastric and intestinal mucosa and the pancreas, to the stage of free amino acids or small peptides. Complete hydrolysis of the latter is effected by intracellular peptidases within the mucosal cells. In any case, free amino acids are the form in which most of the protein nitrogen of the diet eventually appears in the portal blood.

In addition to dietary protein, much protein of endogenous origin appears in the gastrointestinal tract, where it is digested along with that derived from the diet. Part of the endogenous protein consists of the enzymes and mucoproteins secreted by the gastric and intestinal mucosal cells and by the pancreas. The rest consists of tissue proteins derived from desquamated mucosal cells; the mucosa is one of the few tissues of the adult organism in which there occurs continuous renewal of cells. Since amino acids liberated by digestion of endogenous (as well as exogenous) proteins are available for the synthesis of secretory or tissue proteins of the gastrointestinal tract and its appendages, it is evident that the elements of a cyclic pathway are present. Although there is disagreement on the exact magnitude of this endogenous turnover, it appears to approximate the daily dietary protein intake.

In addition to the activities mentioned above, the intestinal mucosa also is engaged in active transport, and, in some cases, significant met-

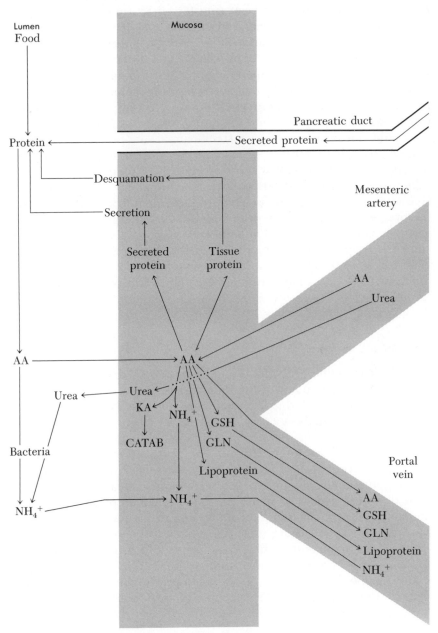

Figure 2–1. Role of gastrointestinal tract in amino acid metabolism.

abolic transformation of amino acids. A fraction of amino acids may be deaminated and their carbon skeletons (alpha-keto acids) catabolized. Even that fraction of amino acids transferred to the portal blood undergoes some alterations. Compared with the pool of amino acids in the intestinal lumen, the amino acids of the portal blood contain much less glutamate and aspartate, but more alanine and glutamine, as well as a significant amount of the tripeptide glutathione (gamma-glutamyl-cysteinyl-glycine) synthesized in the mucosal cells for some as yet unknown reason. The intestinal mucosa also synthesizes certain low-density lipoproteins, which are passed into the portal blood.

In the normal (i.e., not germ-free) mammal, intestinal bacteria play a significant role in nitrogen metabolism. In addition to the production of certain amines, some of which may be toxic or otherwise physiologically active, intestinal bacteria can deaminate amino acids, producing free ammonia. Bacterial urease also produces ammonia by hydrolysis of the urea which is omnipresent in body fluids and hence occurs in the gastrointestinal secretions. The ammonia which is absorbed from the lumen is transported in the portal blood to the liver for detoxication, chiefly by resynthesis of urea. It has been estimated that approximately one-fourth of the daily urea production undergoes this intestinal recycling.

Liver (Fig. 2-2)

The liver is one of the most important sites of amino acid metabolism, from the standpoint of the wide variety of reactions taking place therein as well as of the quantitative significance of many of these processes. In the anabolic direction, liver is the site of synthesis of most of the plasma proteins (the exceptions being the immunoglobulins), of the nonessential* amino acids from keto acids derived from carbohydrate, and of certain special products which are used in the liver or elsewhere (glutathione, glutamine, taurine, carnosine, creatine). In the catabolic direction, liver is the chief site of deamination of amino acids to ammonia and keto acids, and of conversion of the former to urea and the latter to carbohydrate (gluconeogenesis) or fatty acid precursors with eventual oxidation of these non-nitrogenous products for energy. Liver also has a great regulatory influence upon the nitrogen economy of the organism, since it is the first organ to process the incoming constituents of the portal blood; this enables it to act as a metabolic buffer.

---

*Essential amino acids are defined as those which cannot be synthesized, from precursors ordinarily present in the diet, at a rate sufficient to satisfy certain criteria in the organism specified, e.g., optimal growth in the young rat or maintenance of nitrogen equilibrium (q.v.) in the adult human.

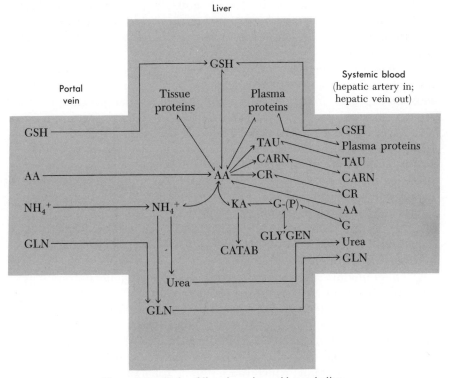

Figure 2–2. Role of liver in amino acid metabolism.

Based upon experiments with dogs fed fairly large meals of protein, it has been concluded that the largest fraction of the free amino acids presented to the liver by the portal blood is catabolized to urea. The next largest fraction is passed on to the systemic circulation as free amino acids, with progressively smaller fractions converted to liver tissue proteins, plasma proteins, and small amounts of special products. In the postabsorptive state all of these processes decrease in rate except the synthesis of plasma proteins, which remains constant.

The liver shares with extrahepatic tissues catabolic pathways for the degradation of nonessential amino acids. Most essential amino acids appear to be degraded exclusively in the liver, except for the branched-chain amino acids (valine, leucine, isoleucine), which are more readily attacked elsewhere.

The deaminated fragments (alpha-keto acids) of most amino acids can be converted to carbohydrate (gluconeogenesis) in the liver, eventually appearing in the liver glycogen or blood glucose. Many of these pathways are reversible, that is, the liver can synthesize nonessential amino acids from waste ammonia and the keto acids derived from carbohydrate catabolism. A smaller group of amino acids produces keto acids

more closely related to the fatty acids and ketone bodies; these fragments cannot produce carbohydrate. In any case, if physiologically
required, all keto acid fragments can be degraded eventually through
the Krebs cycle.

It has been estimated that the liver is responsible for less than half of
the plasma proteins which are catabolized per day. Since the remainder
must be degraded in the periphery, it is quite likely that plasma proteins,
along with their many other functions, should be regarded as an export-
able form of temporarily bound amino acids transported, along with
free amino acids, from the liver to the extrahepatic tissues.

In addition to utilization of the free amino acid pool for synthesis of
proteins, the liver also synthesizes (or passes on from the portal blood)
glutathione and glutamine, varying the output according to physiological conditions. Also produced by the liver, primarily for use in muscle, are taurine (aminoethylsulfonate, from cysteine), carnosine (beta-
alanylhistidine), and creatine (N-methylguanidoacetate, from arginine,
glycine, and methionine).

The ammonia of the portal blood, which incidentally differentiates
this fluid from systemic blood (where only traces of this cytotoxic substance can be detected), is almost entirely converted by the liver to urea,
the chief waste product of amino acid metabolism. Ammonia arising
from deamination of amino acids in the liver undergoes the same conversion. Small quantities of ammonia alternatively may be detoxified by
formation of glutamine, which is a nontoxic form of ammonia, suitable
for transport in the systemic blood to the kidney, where it functions as
a source of urinary ammonia.

Skeletal Muscle (Fig. 2-3)

Although reactions of amino acid metabolism in muscle sometimes
take place at a much slower rate than in liver, the sheer mass of skeletal
muscle makes this tissue quantitatively the most important in the mammalian organism in certain aspects of nitrogen metabolism. This is true,
for example, in the cases of protein synthesis and degradation, creatine
metabolism, and catabolism of the branched-chain amino acids.

Depending upon physiological needs, muscle either takes up or contributes to the free amino acids of plasma. Whether the plasma proteins
can be degraded in muscle remains unknown, but as indicated earlier,
the lack of information on the site of at least one-half of this process still
leaves skeletal muscle as a possible candidate. In any case, the pool of
free amino acids in muscle is in dynamic interaction with a mass of tissue
protein so large that, although much less labile in rate of turnover than
certain other tissues, it makes a major contribution to the economy of the
body when called upon under conditions of protein deprivation.

Muscle contains enzyme systems catalyzing the degradation of
nonessential and, for some as yet unexplained reason, the essential

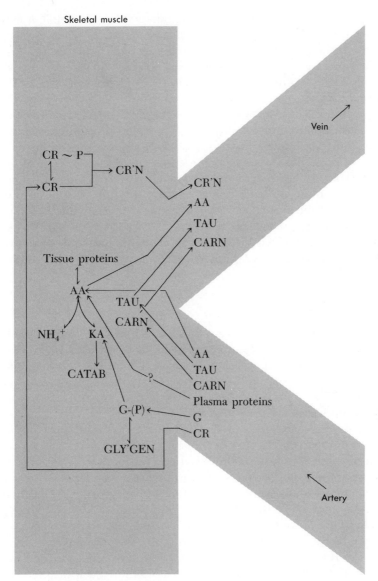

Figure 2–3. Role of skeletal muscle in amino acid metabolism.

branched-chain amino acids. In contrast to liver and (as will be discussed shortly) kidney, the keto acids derived from deamination of amino acids in muscle do not form carbohydrate; i.e., gluconeogenesis is not a significant process in this tissue. The converse reaction, however, can occur: certain nonessential amino acids can be synthesized from keto acids provided by carbohydrate.

Although the metabolism of ammonia in muscle belongs largely to the province of purines and will not be pursued here in detail, it may be noted that the major source of ammonia is adenylate, which is deaminated to inosinate by adenylate deaminase. Adenylate arises during muscle contraction from the operation of the myokinase reaction, which converts ADP (produced from ATP in the muscle twitch) to ATP and adenylate (AMP).

Taurine, carnosine, and anserine (the carnosine analog containing 1-methyl-histidine) are present in high concentration in muscle. Their functions are unknown. 3-Methyl-histidine, which is found in the free state in muscle, also occurs in peptide linkage in actin and myosin.

The role of phosphocreatine as an energy store is too well known to require repetition here. The high concentration of creatine in muscle and the size of the muscle mass underlie the proportionality which is observed between the musculature of an individual and his daily excretion of creatinine, the waste product derived from the spontaneous dehydration of creatine and cyclodephosphorylation of phosphocreatine.

Kidney (Fig. 2-4)

Considering first the role of the kidney in the disposal of nitrogenous waste, it may be noted that its function with regard to the chief waste product, urea, is rather passive. Urea is filtered through the glomerular membrane and, just as mechanically, is partly reabsorbed along with water in the tubules and partly excreted in the urine. The daily output varies with the intake of dietary protein.

Creatinine, since it is not reabsorbed by the tubules, is completely excreted in the urine. In some mammals (including man) tubular secretion occurs also. The amount excreted per day tends to be constant for a given individual (see previous section), provided no drastic alterations are made in the daily consumption of meat, which naturally would contain large amounts of the precursor, creatine.

The daily output of ammonia is related only indirectly to amino acid metabolism, since it correlates primarily with the state of acid-base balance in the organism (see Chapter 5). Amino acids provide the raw material, nevertheless. The major source of ammonia appears to be the amide nitrogen of glutamine, which is synthesized in extrarenal tissues (e.g., liver) and transported in the blood to the kidney, where it is hydrolyzed. A second source is provided by direct deamination of amino acids in the kidney, the resultant keto acids being utilized chiefly for gluconeogenesis, a pathway to which the kidney makes a significant contribution, although it is secondary to the liver in this regard.

Excretion by the kidney of urate, also a nitrogenous waste product, will be mentioned at this point solely for the sake of completeness, since it derives from the pathway of purine catabolism in mammals.

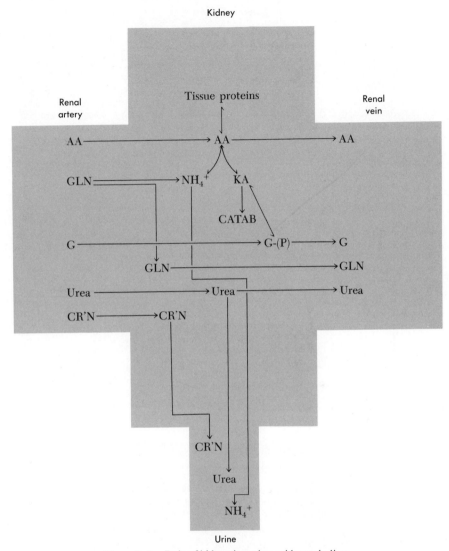

Figure 2-4. Role of kidney in amino acid metabolism.

INTEGRATED REGULATORY SCHEME (Fig. 2-5)

An interesting interrelationship exists between the effects which various regulatory factors have upon overall amino acid metabolism in the body and upon the translocation of amino acids from one group of tissues to another. The mass of skeletal muscle so far exceeds that of other tissues that, although the rate of turnover of the average muscle

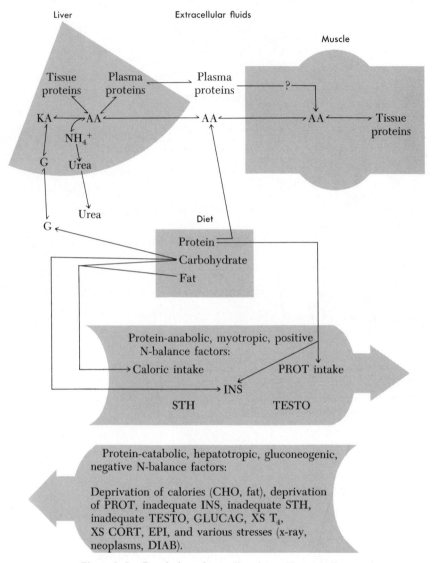

Figure 2–5. Regulation of overall amino acid metabolism.

protein is slow compared with, for example, liver, muscle must be considered the major site of protein synthesis for the entire body. On the other hand, so many of the catabolic pathways for amino acids, particularly those leading to the formation of the waste product urea and carbohydrate (gluconeogenesis), are localized in liver, that this organ must be considered the major catabolic site for the body. In accord with these statements, most protein-anabolic factors also tend to favor the translocation of amino acids from liver (and other visceral organs) to skeletal muscle (and other peripheral tissues of the carcass), hence they may be called *myotropic*. Protein-catabolic, gluconeogenic factors, operating in the opposite direction, therefore can be called *hepatotropic*. (As will be discussed in later chapters, the phenomenon of gluconeogenesis, although it has received the most emphasis in the past, is only one of a concerted group of transformations which takes place upon mobilization of amino acids to the liver from the periphery.)

Anabolic-Myotropic Factors

Positive nitrogen balance,* protein synthesis (particularly in muscle), and translocation of amino acids from liver to muscle are favored by overall caloric intake in the diet (primarily fat and carbohydrate), dietary protein, and the hormones insulin, STH (somatotropic or growth hormone), and testosterone.

Fat and carbohydrate share a rather nonspecific caloric effect (so, for that matter, does alcohol), presumably based largely on the ability of these fuels to sustain the energy requirements of the body, thus obviating the need to degrade amino acids for this purpose. In addition to this rather simple mechanism of protein-sparing, carbohydrate alone exhibits certain more sophisticated effects, such as protein-sparing on a protein-inadequate diet, which fat does not. These qualities of carbohydrate probably are due, in part, to the ability of this substance (not shared with fat) to provide carbon skeletons (alpha-keto acids) for synthesis of nonessential amino acids, plus the well-established stimulus which carbohydrate gives to the secretion of insulin, the effects of which are discussed below.

Dietary protein provides not only the raw material for protein anabolism in the body (amino acids) but also the postprandial rise in plasma amino acids which acts as a stimulus (along with glucose) for secretion of insulin.

Insulin, secreted in response to a rise in plasma glucose and/or amino acids, causes deposition of amino acids in skeletal muscle and their incorporation into muscle protein. Growth hormone and androgens (primarily testosterone) also promote these effects, probably independently of insulin, although in some test systems the presence of insulin is required for the other hormones to be effective.

Thyroid hormones are required, in physiological amounts, for growth and differentiation in the young, although the major effect of these hormones (in excess) is catabolic, as discussed on following page.

---

*Nitrogen balance is defined as the difference between the nitrogen intake (food) and output (primarily urinary and fecal N) per day. It is positive in growth and pregnancy, negative in wasting diseases and conditions of protein loss, and zero (N equilibrium) in the normal adult. More detailed discussions can be found in textbooks of biochemistry.

Catabolic-Hepatotropic Factors

Negative nitrogen balance, protein catabolism (chiefly in muscle), amino-acid catabolism and gluconeogenesis (chiefly in liver), and translocation of amino acids from skeletal muscle to liver are favored by deprivation of calories or protein, inadequacy of insulin or growth hormone or testosterone, excessive amounts of thyroid hormones, glucagon, and glucocorticoid hormones and those factors stimulating their secretion (ACTH, epinephrine, irradiation, tumors, and various other forms of stress).

A diet inadequate in caloric content, even though adequate in protein, will result in negative nitrogen balance, as will a diet deficient in protein but adequate calorically. Per weight of tissue, wastage of body protein in these cases is felt most severely by those tissues with the greatest rate of turnover of protein, namely gastrointestinal mucosa, liver, kidney, and pancreas. On the other hand, the greatest total loss of protein is suffered by muscle, since its mass more than compensates for its lower rate of turnover. The nitrogen lost from muscle (and other tissues) in these conditions of dietary deprivation appears largely as urea in the urine, derived from hepatic deamination of those amino acids which are endogenous to the liver, or arise from the degradation of liver protein, or are brought in the blood from the catabolism of protein in peripheral tissues (e.g., muscle). Some of the keto acids resulting as by-products eventually appear as blood glucose (gluconeogenesis) or are converted to fragments which are oxidized via the Krebs cycle.

Similar shifts of amino acid metabolism toward a predominantly catabolic direction and toward the liver are produced by deficiencies of the anabolic hormones (insulin, STH, and testosterone) and in hyperthyroid conditions, in which the breakdown of most of the organic metabolites of the body appears to be accelerated rather nonspecifically.

Certain hormones function specifically as protein-catabolic agents, namely glucagon and the glucocorticoids. It must be noted in this connection, however, that such a categorization refers to the overall effect which these hormones have upon the nitrogen economy of the body. In terms of certain proteins, specifically a number of hepatic enzymes, the action of glucagon and the glucocorticoids is definitely anabolic.

The catecholamines (epinephrine, norepinephrine) sometimes are listed along with the protein-catabolic hormones. As neurotransmitters in the sympathetic nervous system and as neurohormones in the general circulation, they are involved in the general response to stress, causing the secretion of ACTH, which in turn causes the secretion of glucocorticoids. Although direct effects upon gluconeogenesis and urea formation in liver have been described, these have required unphysiological concentrations. Hence, in all probability, the catecholamines function in this respect indirectly, as indicated above.

Protein-Caloric Deprivation in Man

In technologically underdeveloped areas of the world the infant, upon partial and later complete cessation of breast-feeding, often is presented with a diet low in calories and protein content, the latter usually also of poor quality (due to the deficiency of essential amino acids, such as lysine, in the cereal proteins offered to the child upon weaning). When the deficiencies in calories and protein are about equally severe, the resultant condition is known as marasmus, characterized by loss of adipose tissue, wasting of muscle protein, and a general appearance of emaciation. Paradoxically, due to its protein-anabolic, myotropic action, the addition of an excessive proportion of carbohydrate (in the form of starchy gruels, cereals, or sugar in sugar cane) to the diet in relation to the content of protein causes the condition of the child to worsen. The translocation of nitrogen from liver to muscle decreases the ability to synthesize plasma proteins, resulting in hypoproteinemia (especially hypoalbuminemia) and edema. Fatty liver also occurs. The total syndrome which thus develops is known as kwashiorkor. As might be expected, all gradations between marasmus and kwashiorkor are seen clinically.

A new regulatory mechanism has come to light in recent years, discovered in the course of starvation therapy of human obesity. Total starvation depletes the glycogen stores in a day or two, after which energy requirements are met, partly by degradation of protein (initially supplied by the metabolically labile tissues such as liver, pancreas, and gastrointestinal tract, and later by skeletal muscle), but mainly by fatty acids mobilized from the adipose depots. These latter stores of energy may be adequate to sustain an average individual for a month or so, and in the grossly obese for many months. Patients on a diet consisting solely of water, minerals, and vitamins adapt to this regimen after a few weeks. Part of this adaptation involves a decrease in the catabolism of protein and in the rate of gluconeogenesis from amino acids. The regulatory mechanism underlying this change is unknown, but has been determined to operate through a decreased rate of release of amino acids from muscle for transport to the liver.

REFERENCES

Role of Individual Organs

Fauconneau, G., and Michel, M. C.: The role of the gastrointestinal tract in the regulation of protein metabolism. *In*: Munro, H. N. (ed.): Mammalian Protein Metabolism. Vol. 4. New York, Academic Press, Inc., 1970, pp. 481-522.

Elwyn, D. H.: The role of the liver in regulation of amino acid and protein metabolism. *In*: Munro, H. N. (ed.): Mammalian Protein Metabolism. Vol. 4. New York, Academic Press, Inc., 1970, pp. 523–557.

Cahill, G. F., Jr., and Owen, O. E.: The role of the kidney in the regulation of protein metabolism. *In*: Munro, H. N. (ed.): Mammalian Protein Metabolism. Vol. 4. New York, Academic Press, Inc., 1970, pp. 559–584.

Young, V. R.: The role of skeletal and cardiac muscle in the regulation of protein metabolism. *In*: Munro, H. N. (ed.): Mammalian Protein Metabolism. Vol. 4. New York, Academic Press, Inc., 1970, pp. 585–674.

Role of Dietary and Hormonal Factors

Leathem, J. H.: Some aspects of hormone and protein metabolic interrelationships. *In*: Munro, H. N., and Allison, J. B. (eds.): Mammalian Protein Metabolism. Vol. 1. New York, Academic Press, Inc., 1964, pp. 343–380.

Munro, H. N.: General aspects of the regulation of protein metabolism by diet and by hormones. *In*: Munro, H. N., and Allison, J. B. (eds.): Mammalian Protein Metabolism. Vol. 1. New York, Academic Press, Inc., 1964, pp. 381–481.

Manchester, K. L.: Sites of hormonal regulation of protein metabolism. *In*: Munro, H. N. (ed.): Mammalian Protein Metabolism. Vol. 4. New York, Academic Press, 1970, pp. 229–298.

Marasmus and Kwashiorkor

Platt, B. S., Heard, C. R. C., and Stewart, R. J. C.: Experimental protein-calorie deficiency. *In*: Munro, H. N., and Allison, J. B. (eds.): Mammalian Protein Metabolism. Vol. 2. New York, Academic Press, Inc., 1964, pp. 445–521.

Viteri, F., Béhar, M., Arroyave, G., and Scrimshaw, N. S.: Clinical aspects of protein malnutrition. *In*: Munro, H. N., and Allison, J. B. (eds): Mammalian Protein Metabolism. Vol. 2. New York, Academic Press, Inc., 1964, pp. 523–568.

Therapeutic Starvation

Marliss, E., Aoki, T. T., Felig, P., Pozefsky, T., and Cahill, G. F., Jr.: Hormones and substrates in the regulation of gluconeogenesis in fasting man. Adv. Enz. Reg. 8:3–11 (1970).

3

AMINO ACID TRANSPORT

The previous chapter discussed the regulation of the mass flow of amino acids among metabolic pathways and among tissues without inquiring into the mechanistic details. Underlying the processes of flow into and out of tissues and into and out of metabolic sequences and cycles, there exist mechanisms of regulation of transport and mechanisms of regulation of enzymes, respectively. This chapter and several which succeed it will be devoted to these more specific topics.

TYPES OF TRANSPORT SYSTEMS (Fig. 3-1)

Passive Diffusion (Fig. 3-1 *A*)

Passive diffusion represents the simplest form of transport through biological membranes and is almost universally present, the more complex forms of transport usually being superimposed upon it. Diffusion proceeds freely in both directions, but *net* flow only from the side of higher to the side of lower concentration (more accurately, activity). In the case of systems handling water-soluble solutes (e.g., amino acids), the effective pore size of the membranes appears to fall in the range of 3.5 to 7.0 Å.

Characteristics of this type of transport include a low temperature coefficient, insensitivity to inhibitors of glycolysis, oxidation or oxidative phosphorylation, absence of competitive effects between compounds of similar structure, and nonsaturability with increasing concentrations of solute.

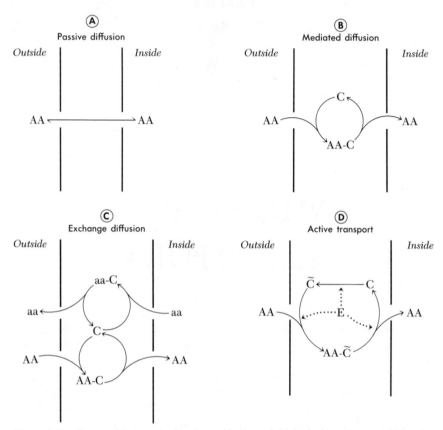

Figure 3–1. Types of transport of amino acids through biological membranes. Abbreviations: AA, aa = amino acids, C = amino-acid carrier, $\tilde{C}$ = activated or otherwise altered form of carrier, E = source of energy.

Mediated Diffusion (Fig. 3-1 *B*)

This type of transport, also called *facilitated diffusion,* shares with the preceding type the characteristic of being "downhill," since it also proceeds along the direction of the concentration gradient. It has one important added feature, a hypothetical carrier of unknown structure, which combines with the amino acid on one side of the membrane, transports it through the membrane, then releases it at the other side. The carrier has been alternatively conceived of as a macromolecule (probably protein) which shuttles back and forth between the two surfaces of the membrane, or as a part of a macromolecule (akin to the prosthetic group of an enzyme) which oscillates back and forth on a stem. Whatever its structure, the carrier exhibits considerable specificity toward the structure of the substance carried.

Being independent of energy input, as is passive diffusion, this type of transport also is insensitive to various metabolic inhibitors. However, it differs from the first type in having a higher temperature coefficient, exhibits the phenomenon of competition between structurally related solutes, and resembles an enzyme in saturability with increasing solute concentration. Its behavior in this last regard, in fact, can be described by the Michaelis-Menten equation. The enzyme-like properties of this and other carrier-containing transport systems has led microbiologists to adopt the infelicitous term *permease* for the analogous mechanisms in the bacterial membrane.

Exchange Diffusion (Fig. 3-1 *C*)

If, in the preceding system, two amino acids can be transported by the same carrier, then the phenomenon of exchange diffusion is possible. Assume that amino acid aa in the figure is present in higher concentration inside than outside the membrane (i.e., the cell is preloaded with aa). The resultant efflux of aa can drive the influx of AA, even though this may be against a concentration gradient. All that is required for the two processes combined is a net decrease in free energy, so that the overall reaction is exergonic, or downhill. The situation is the same in many bioenergetic systems, where an exergonic reaction drives an endergonic reaction, the two being coupled through a common intermediary. Looking at the system mechanistically rather than thermodynamically, the efflux of aa can be regarded as bringing the carrier into contact with AA more frequently than would otherwise occur.

Active Transport (Fig. 3-1 *D*)

Whereas in the preceding example uphill transport was driven by downhill transport, in the type now under consideration, uphill transport is driven by the metabolic energy of the cell. Consequently, it is sensitive to metabolic inhibitors. Since it involves a carrier, it shares the characteristics noted for the preceding carrier-containing systems, namely a relatively high temperature coefficient, competition between solutes, and saturability.

Evidence from a number of tissues indicates that, within a given tissue, the same carrier is involved in mediated, exchange, and active transport of a given solute or family of solutes. Although the figure portrays the carrier in two forms, one activated, the actual site of the expenditure of energy is unknown. It may well be that energy is utilized in converting the carrier to a high-energy form which is more readily able to combine with the amino acid at the outer surfaces. Other possibilities are activation of the amino acid, activation of the combination reaction of amino acid plus carrier, and activation of the dissociation reaction at the other surface of the membrane. Depending upon the type of cell, energy for the activation may come from aerobic oxidations or from glycolysis.

AMINO ACID TRANSPORT GROUPS (Fig. 3-2)

Although the specificity of the carrier alluded to in previous sections sometimes is quite narrow, being restricted to one or two compounds, generally a carrier handles a family or group of amino acids of similar structure. It is also not unusual to find that certain amino acids, although transported chiefly by one carrier system, also participate in other systems to a greater or lesser extent. (Amino acids of the D configuration, having no great significance in mammalian metabolism, will merely be

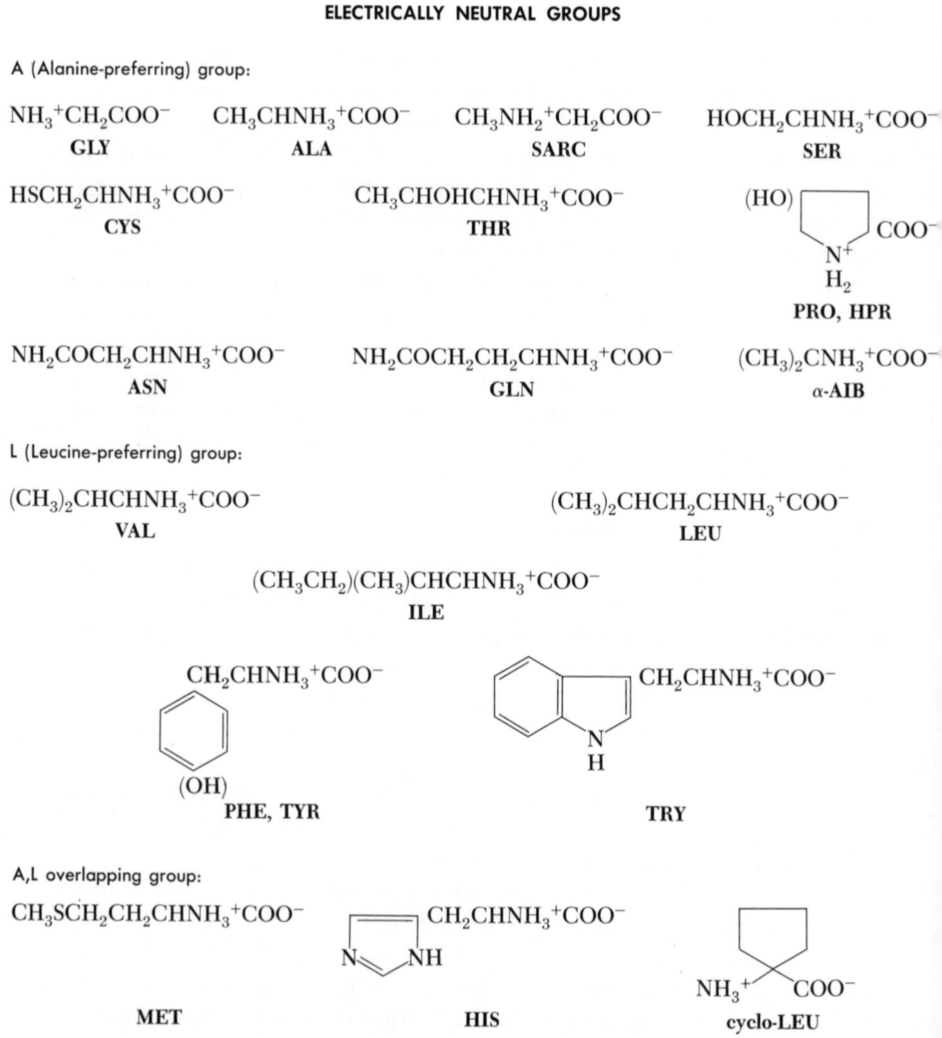

ELECTRICALLY NEUTRAL GROUPS

A (Alanine-preferring) group:

$NH_3{}^+CH_2COO^-$ $CH_3CHNH_3{}^+COO^-$ $CH_3NH_2{}^+CH_2COO^-$ $HOCH_2CHNH_3{}^+COO^-$
    GLY   ALA   SARC   SER

$HSCH_2CHNH_3{}^+COO^-$ $CH_3CHOHCHNH_3{}^+COO^-$ (HO)
    CYS   THR

PRO, HPR

$NH_2COCH_2CHNH_3{}^+COO^-$ $NH_2COCH_2CH_2CHNH_3{}^+COO^-$ $(CH_3)_2CNH_3{}^+COO^-$
    ASN   GLN   α-AIB

L (Leucine-preferring) group:

$(CH_3)_2CHCHNH_3{}^+COO^-$ $(CH_3)_2CHCH_2CHNH_3{}^+COO^-$
    VAL   LEU

$(CH_3CH_2)(CH_3)CHCHNH_3{}^+COO^-$
    ILE

$CH_2CHNH_3{}^+COO^-$ $CH_2CHNH_3{}^+COO^-$

(OH)
   PHE, TYR   TRY

A,L overlapping group:

$CH_3SCH_2CH_2CHNH_3{}^+COO^-$ $CH_2CHNH_3{}^+COO^-$

$NH_3{}^+ \quad COO^-$

    MET   HIS   cyclo-LEU

Figure 3–2. Structural transport groups of amino acids.

Illustration continued on opposite page

mentioned in passing. They are frequently actively, but much more slowly, transported by the same systems as their L isomers.)

Complete surveys of amino acid transport groups have been made in relatively few tissues. Nevertheless, it appears that most tissues contain the same or very similar systems. Major differences, where they occur, can be ascribed to the metabolic needs or peculiarities of individual tissues. These will be pointed out in subsequent sections.

All types of cells contain transport systems for the electrically neutral amino acids, and in most cells, this large group is subdivided further. One common division separates the smaller and more polar amino acids (the A or alanine-preferring system) from those with larger and more hydrophobic side chains (the L or leucine-preferring system). Although carried preferentially by one system or the other, most amino acids in either group are transported, but less efficiently, by the other system.

Iminoglycine group:

$NH_3^+CH_2COO^-$ $CH_3NH_2^+CH_2COO^-$ $(CH_3)_2NH^+CH_2COO^-$ $(CH_3)_3N^+CH_2COO^-$
     GLY   **SARC**   **Dimethyl-GLY**   **Betaine**

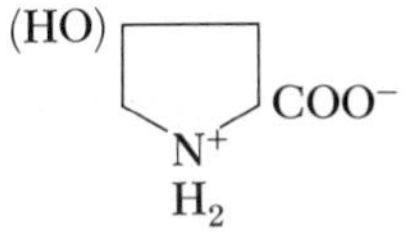

PRO, HPR

β-Amino group:

$NH_3^+CH_2CH_2COO^-$ $NH_3^+CH_2CH_2SO_3^-$ $(NH_3^+CH_2)(CH_3)CHCOO^-$
   β-ALA   **TAU**   **β-AIB**

Guanidino group:

$NH_2^+:CNH_2(CH_3)NCH_2COO^-$
       CR

ANIONIC GROUP

$^-OOCCH_2CHNH_3^+COO^-$ $^-OOCCH_2CH_2CHNH_3^+COO^-$
   ASP   **GLU**

CATIONIC (LYS⁺) GROUP PLUS CYSTINE

$NH_2^+:CNH_2NHCH_2CH_2CH_2CHNH_3^+COO^-$ $NH_3^+CH_2CH_2CH_2CH_2CHNH_3^+COO^-$
       ARG   **LYS**

$NH_3^+CH_2CH_2CH_2CHNH_3^+COO^-$ $^-OOCCHNH_3^+CH_2SSCH_2CHNH_3^+COO^-$
    ORN   **(CYS)₂**

Figure 3–2. *Continued.*

Methionine and histidine are transported equally well by both systems, at least in the Ehrlich ascites cell, where much of this classificatory work was done, and hence are tabulated here as A, L, overlapping.

Investigations of amino-acid transport frequently are hampered by metabolic alterations undergone by an amino acid once it enters a cell. Artificial, nonmetabolizable, model amino acids have been of great help in circumventing this problem. Two which are widely used are shown in Figure 3-2: alpha-aminoisobutyrate (AIB) which is transported with the A group, and 1-aminocyclopentane-1-carboxylate (cycloleucine) which belongs to the completely overlapping group. These amino acids not only are transported as are natural compounds but also are amenable to the same regulatory influences (e.g., hormones).

In addition to the two groups mentioned, many tissues contain transport systems for the iminoglycine or betaine group (glycine and its methylated derivatives as well as the imino acids) and the beta-amino group (possibly including also gamma-aminobutyrate) among the neutral amino acids, as well as systems for anionic and for cationic (diamino) amino acids. More restricted in distribution is a system for transport of guanidino compounds.

EFFLUX SYSTEMS

Most of the investigations of transport of amino acids across biological membranes have been concerned with flux into the cell; efflux has been studied much less extensively. Apparently many amino acids leave the cell by the same mechanism through which they enter, sometimes by carrier-mediated or exchange diffusion, sometimes by active transport, the influx systems simply operating in reverse for efflux. In certain cases, however, the characteristics for the efflux system of a particular amino acid are quite different from those of the system for influx.

CHARACTERISTICS OF SELECTED TISSUES

Intestine

Transport systems of the neutral (not yet differentiated into the A and L subgroups), iminoglycine, and diamino types have been reported. The anionic system may well be present also, but its detection is made difficult by the extensive transamination undergone by aspartate and glutamate during absorption.

A question on the true specificity of amino acid carriers is raised by the observation (in kidney as well as intestine) that hexoses compete with the transport of certain amino acids. In addition, a relationship is suggested with the transport systems for inorganic cations, since many of the amino acid transport systems are functional only in the presence of Na^+ ions outside the membrane. Na^+ ions have been shown to accompany the amino acid across the membrane in many instances, and the amino acid as well as the Na^+ transfer is inhibited by ouabain, which characteristically blocks the action of the so-called sodium-potassium activated transport ATPases. Further information on this last topic can be found in the monograph, *Physiological Chemistry of Lipids in Mammals* in this series.

An inborn error of transport of the neutral amino acids (groups A and L) occurs in the intestine (as well as in the kidney) in Hartnup disease. Most of the pellagra-like symptoms are referable to the deficiency of tryptophan, one metabolic pathway of which normally leads to the formation of the vitamin nicotinamide.

Cystinuria originally was believed to be an inborn error of the intermediary metabolism of cystine or cysteine. When cystine in the urine was found to be accompanied by lysine, arginine, and ornithine, an inborn error of transport was postulated, affecting diamino acids, although cystine differed from the others in the group by its electrical neutrality at physiological pH. Strong supporting evidence for the transport defect came from the discovery of cystinurics whose *intestinal* (as well as renal) absorption of the entire group of diamino acids was deficient. However, the situation has become more complex in recent years with the recognition of three different types of cystinuria and a noncystinuric hyperdiaminoaciduria, the varying patterns of intestinal absorption and renal reabsorption requiring the recognition of separate systems of transport for cystine on the one hand and for lysine, arginine, and ornithine on the other. It has been suggested that, in intestine at least, cystine is absorbed by two mechanisms, one specific for itself, and one shared with the cationic amino acids. The cystine problem will be discussed further in connection with transport in the kidney.

Kidney*

It is believed that the kidney possesses separate transport systems for the following groups of amino acids: neutral (probably subdivided into A and L types), iminoglycine, beta-amino, cationic, and anionic. As in the case of intestine, hexoses interfere with amino acid transport in kidney. Likewise, dependence upon the presence of Na^+ has been reported.

As mentioned previously, renal reabsorption of neutral amino acids is defective in the inborn error, Hartnup disease.

In addition to the iminoglycine system, which has been character-

---

*Meister (Science *180*:33–39, 1973) has cited evidence for the participation of a *gamma-glutamyl* cycle in amino acid transport in kidney (and probably other tissues), with glutathione serving as glutamyl-donor to the transported amino acid.

ized as a low-affinity, high-capacity type, there is evidence in kidney for discrete systems carrying glycine and the prolines. These more specific systems have high affinity and low capacity for substrates. The inborn error hyperiminoglycinuria affects the first-mentioned common system, whereas glycine alone is excreted in another genetically transmitted renal defect.

Some of the complexities which characterize the transport of the cationic amino acids and cystine have been indicated in the section on intestine. Differences do exist between the two tissues. Biopsy samples of at least some cystinurics have shown definite competition for transport between cystine and the cationic amino acids in the intestine as well as a marked deficiency in the transport of cystine as such. In contrast, although kidney samples from cystinurics exhibit a deficiency in the transport of cationic amino acids and competition within this group (also shown in normal kidney), there is no indication that cystine shares this system. Consequently, the excretion of cystine along with the cationic amino acids in cystinuria seems inexplicable.

Once it reaches an intracellular destination, cystine is largely reduced to cysteine, which is known to be transported across membranes by a system different from that utilized by cystine. Of possible significance in connection with attempts to explain the findings in cystinuria are reports that the *efflux* of cysteine from kidney cortex cells is inhibited by the cationic amino acids. Since cysteine and cystine are in oxidation-reduction equilibrium with each other in the cell, it is possible that, in cystinuria, the cationic amino acids inhibit the excretion of cysteine, which builds up in concentration in the cells, leading to the formation and excretion of excessive amounts of cystine, even though the inborn error is not directly connected with the latter compound in the kidney.

Liver

Despite its prime importance as a site of intense metabolism of amino acids, little is known of the transport mechanisms in liver. Using a nonmetabolizable amino acid (AIB), liver slices have been shown to contain a system which concentrates amino acids linearly with time; is saturable with substrate; inhibited by anoxia, dinitrophenol (an uncoupling agent for oxidative generation of energy), and ouabain; and requires Na^+ as well as K^+ and Ca^{++}. Cycloleucine, which is much bulkier in structure, is transported less efficiently.

The concentration of AIB by rat liver slices is inhibited by glycine, which itself is actively transported. Cystine is transported by a mechanism which is inhibited by glycine, but not by AIB. On the other hand, the related amino acid, cysteine, is transported by two systems, one of high and one of low affinity, both inhibited by glycine, but only the high-affinity system by AIB (weakly).

Brain

The systems reported for active transport of amino acids in brain slices may not have much physiological significance *in vivo* because of the blood-brain barrier. *In vivo* transport is said to resemble the mediated rather than the active type. Whatever their ultimate evaluation, brain slices have been reported to contain separate systems for the transport of the following amino acid groups: neutral (divisible into A and L types), beta-amino (including gamma-amino), cationic, and anionic. DOPA (dihydroxyphenylalanine) shares the same carrier as other aromatic amino acids (presumably the L system). Carnosine, creatine, ethanolamine, and choline also are actively transported.

Muscle

As in the case of liver, little is known of specific transport systems for amino acids in muscle. Even in the case of the regulatory studies which will be discussed in a later section, little attention has been paid to amino acids of different structural types, and most investigators have used diaphragm, or occasionally heart, rather than skeletal muscle, which is the preponderant muscle mass of the body.

Skeletal muscle contains a specific transport system for creatine. Of other guanidino compounds tested, only beta-guanidinopropionate is transported, although the system can be inhibited by guanidinoacetate and a few other compounds of similar structure.

Blood Cells

Reticulocytes of many species and avian erythrocytes (which retain much of their metabolic machinery even when mature) contain many of the systems for amino-acid transport already described, such as neutral (A and L types), iminoglycine, and beta-amino. The mature mammalian erythrocyte, on the other hand, is limited largely to the L system, and this appears to function by way of mediated rather than active transport.

Anaerobic glycolysis furnishes the energy for active transport in leukocytes, which appear to contain systems for several types of amino acids. It is of interest that, in cystinurics, there is no defect in the leukocytic transport systems for cationic amino acids or for cystine.

Ehrlich Ascites Tumor Cells

Although not a normal tissue, so much of the pioneer work on mechanisms of transport of amino acids has been and is being done with ascites cells, that a brief review of their properties in this regard may not be out of order.

Ehrlich ascites tumor cells contain most of the systems already described. As a matter of fact, many of these systems were first detected and characterized in ascites cells, including the neutral A and L types, the beta-amino, and the cationic. No iminoglycine system is present. Ascites cells contain an ASC (alanine, serine, cysteine) system, which also transports proline, and is said to be found also in reticulocytes and avian erythrocytes.

The A system is Na^+-dependent, one Na^+ molecule migrating into the cell per amino acid molecule. It is more sensitive than the L system toward temperature and pH, its activity becoming negligible at pH 5. Little exchange-diffusion is shown by this system. Its specificity toward chain length in solutes shows two maxima, one at the size of alanine, the second at the size of methionine. It is more sensitive than the L system toward anoxia and respiratory inhibitors.

In contrast, the L system of ascites cells is little affected by Na^+ or pH, is less temperature-sensitive and exhibits strong activity in exchange-diffusion. Its affinity is poor for chain lengths less than five carbon atoms.

The beta-amino system resembles the A system in its Na^+ requirements, as does the ASC system. Exchange-diffusion has not been detected in the beta-amino system and is weak in the ASC system. The latter is only moderately sensitive to pH.

The cationic system is Na^+-dependent in ascites cells (but may be independent in leukocytes). At low pH, when it bears a net positive charge, histidine can be carried by the cationic system. Neutral amino acids of the L group, if of proper structure, also can be transported along with sodium, the Na^+ occupying a position corresponding to that of the positively charged second ammonium-type group in the amino acids normally carried by the cationic system.

The nonsaturable component of transport of many amino acids has been assumed to be simple, passive diffusion, as indicated earlier. Experiments with ascites and a few other types of cells suggest that the diffusion may not be altogether simple. For example, there is evidence of some degree of structural specificity, and sensitivity to pH and temperature.

REGULATION OF AMINO ACID TRANSPORT (Table 3-1)

Most of the known regulatory factors in transport of amino acids are endocrine in nature, a fact which poses certain problems in the compilation and interpretation of data such as are collected in Table 3-1. As is the case in most hormonal effects, two virtually opposing factors lurk behind the designs of the quoted experiments, namely, specificity on the one hand, and physiological significance on the other. Proceeding from the most physiological to the most specific situation, a hormone

Table 3–1. *Effects of Regulatory Factors on Transport of Amino Acids*

REGULATORY FACTOR	TARGET TISSUE(S)	EFFECT ON TRANSPORT	NOTES
Growth hormone (STH)	Skeletal muscle, liver, intestine, kidney, heart, adipose, diaphragm	+	Said to affect chiefly the A system
Insulin	Skeletal muscle, liver, heart, diaphragm, adrenal, thyroid, fetal bone	+	Said to affect chiefly the A system
Thyroid hormones	Cartilage, embryonic bone Pituitary, intestine	+ −	Said to affect chiefly the L system
Glucocorticoids	Liver Diaphragm, thymus, spleen, HeLa (and other cultured cells)	+ −	
cAMP	Liver, kidney, embryonic bone, uterus, isolated thyroid cells	+	May be mediator for several hormones; may circulate; affects most transport systems
Glucagon	Liver	+	Probably functions via cAMP
Epinephrine	Heart, liver, kidney, intestine Diaphragm, adipose	+ −	May function via cAMP
Estrogens	Uterus, ascites cells	+	Said to affect chiefly the A system; reported to decrease renal tubular reabsorption
Androgens	Skeletal muscle, kidney, uterus, prostate, seminal vesicle, levator ani	+	Reported also to increase renal tubular reabsorption
Parathyroid hormone (PTH)	Bone, kidney	+	Probably functions via cAMP
Adrenocorticotropic hormone (ACTH)	Adrenals	+	Reported also to decrease renal tubular reabsorption
Thyrotropic hormone (TSH)	Thyroid, skeletal muscle, liver	+	Action on iodide transport via cAMP
Follicle-stimulating hormone (FSH)	Ovary	+	
High-protein diet	Liver	+	Probably via increased glucagon and cAMP
Avitaminosis E	Skeletal muscle, diaphragm	+	
Avitaminosis B$_6$	Intestine, ascites cells, kidney, heart, skeletal muscle	−	Probably via decreased STH secretion
Growth, development	Liver, kidney, other tissues	Variable	See text for details

may be injected into an intact animal (or a deficiency may be produced by surgical excision or pharmacological blockage) and the rate of uptake of an amino acid (preferably isotopically labeled) determined *in vivo* by assay of the tissue concerned after sacrifice of the animal (or perhaps by biopsy sample). A mixed *in vivo—in vitro* design may be used, pre-treating the animal with hormone as described, but then assaying the rate of uptake of amino acid in an *in vitro* tissue preparation, such as a perfused organ or slices of tissue. A completely *in vitro* procedure would involve use of an isolated tissue preparation, both in the exposure to the hormone and to the amino acid being tested.

The first two designs carry with them the danger that the observed effects may be indirect and due to some secondary influence produced by the administered hormone. The last design, although the most specific, frequently is open to the criticism of not being physiological, since it is sometimes difficult to demonstrate any significant effects unless the hormone in question is present at higher than physiological concentrations. It must be admitted also that, in both the second and third examples given, the tissue is not in its normal milieu at the time the transport of the amino acid is taking place. The foregoing considerations should be kept in mind during the following discussion. (Table 3-1 does not distinguish between *in vivo* and *in vitro* techniques; in cases of conflicting reports, the most reasonable and consistent have been selected.)

Hormones with General Anabolic Effects

GROWTH HORMONE.   Although growth hormone facilitates transport of amino acids in most tissues tested, the predominance of the skeletal muscle mass results in a net translocation of nitrogen from visceral organs to muscle (myotropic influence). The positive influence on protein synthesis probably aids in this effect, although the two actions of the hormone are independent of each other.

It has been suggested that the action of growth hormone is restricted to the A group of amino acids; effects on compounds of the L group are explained by lack of strict specificity of the carrier system.

Since an acceleration of the transport of amino acids into diaphragm *in vitro* is detectable after 10 to 15 minutes of incubation with growth hormone, it is probable that no major amount of protein synthesis is required as part of the mechanism of action of the hormone. Nevertheless, participation of a protein in the system is indicated by the fact that prolonged preincubation with inhibitors of protein synthesis abolishes the subsequent effect of growth hormone.

Growth-promoting factors, probably polypeptides, which can be extracted from calf muscle, increase the uptake of leucine and AIB by diaphragm. It is suggested that these substances may be mediators for the action of growth hormone.

As will be discussed in a later section, the effect of avitaminosis B_6 on transport probably manifests itself through a deficiency of growth hormone.

INSULIN.   Since insulin, like growth hormone, favors entry of amino acids into most tissues, its influence in a generally myotropic direction requires the same explanation as that used in the previous case. Insulin also may be specific for amino acids of the A group.

Despite these similarities, there is considerable evidence that the two hormones act upon the transport system independently: (a) the action of growth hormone is not blocked by experimental diabetes; (b) the effect of insulin on the diaphragm *in vitro* is evident in 5 minutes, rather than the minimum of 10 to 15 minutes required by growth hormone; and (c) inhibition of the insulin effect in diaphragm by preincubation with inhibitors of protein synthesis requires much longer times than with growth hormone.

Investigation has shown the existence of at least four routes for the uptake of alanine by diaphragm. One is nonsaturable, presumably representing simple diffusion; this accounts for one-fourth of the total transport. Of the three saturable routes, one is independent of the presence of Na^+ and may well be a demonstration of the overlapping specificity of the L system for alanine. One of the two Na^+-dependent routes is insensitive to insulin; it is suggested that this may be the ASC system. The final route is Na^+-dependent and insulin-sensitive but accounts for no more than 15 per cent of the total saturable transport of alanine. Results such as these serve to emphasize that endocrine regulators generally do not, of themselves, initiate or terminate whole metabolic or translocational pathways, but rather modulate those which are already present.

Paradoxically, transport of amino acids is increased in experimental diabetes. Evidently the massive hepatotropic translocation of nitrogen and negative nitrogen balance observed in this condition are due to factors other than the influence of lack of insulin on amino acid transport.

Recent reports indicate that, in addition to ordinary amino acids, insulin may also facilitate uptake of creatine by skeletal muscle.

ANDROGENS. Gonadal hormones may be expected to exert their primary effects upon those tissues directly concerned with the sex of the organism, and, consequently, will be discussed later in this chapter under Hormones with Specialized Metabolic Effects. Testosterone and a few other androgens, however, possess in addition true general protein-anabolic properties, both in favoring protein synthesis and in transport of amino acids in skeletal muscle. Androgens also exert unexplained growth-promoting effects on the kidney (renotropic effects); perhaps related to this is the reported positive influence on renal tubular reabsorption of amino acids.

Hormones with General Catabolic Effects

THYROID HORMONES. Although thyroxine and related hormones exhibit a positive effect on transport in certain tissues and a negative effect in others, their general catabolic influence in the organism as a whole (when present in excess) may be attributed to an acceleration of the rate of protein degradation. In contrast to growth hormone and insulin, thyroid hormones are said to influence the transport chiefly of the L group of amino acids. The negative effect on pituitary may be related to the feedback mechanism by which the output of thyrotropic hormone is controlled by the amount of circulating thyroid hormones.

GLUCOCORTICOIDS.   At least part of the protein-catabolic action of glucocorticoid hormones is explicable by their effects on transport. By increasing amino acid transport into liver and decreasing it in diaphragm and other tissues, nitrogen translocation in a hepatotropic sense is certainly favored. Investigations of skeletal muscle have shown little or no effect of these hormones upon amino acid transport systems directly. However, by inhibiting protein synthesis in muscle, the glucocorticoids cause an expansion of the intracellular pool of free amino acids, which of itself will augment the rate of efflux into the body fluids.

Glucocorticoids have an inhibitory effect on transport of amino acids into diaphragm *in vitro*, but only after several hours of preincubation. This lag, as well as several other characteristics of the system, have led investigators to conclude that the hormones are inhibiting synthesis of a protein. Possibly relevant to these results are recent reports that glucocorticoids induce alterations in the surface membrane of hepatoma cells in culture, reflected in changes in electrophoretic behavior, antigenicity, and adhesiveness. This induction has a lag period of several hours, and again, there is evidence that synthesis of a protein is involved.

CYCLIC AMP.   Although not considered a hormone in the strict sense, cAMP is listed separately here, since it acts as the second messenger for several of the hormones which follow, a number of investigations have employed it *in vitro*, and finally, its appearance in the circulating body fluids may not be entirely adventitious.

It has been reported that preincubation with cAMP (of the order of 1 hour or so) stimulates uptake of amino acids by liver, kidney, and embryonic bone. Although there is some disagreement in the literature, neutral amino acids of both A and L transport groups seem to be affected. A protein (carrier?) essential to the stimulation of transport probably is synthesized during the preincubation.

More recent investigations have extended the effects of cAMP to uterus and isolated thyroid cells, and, in kidney slices, have demonstrated the participation of amino acids from the A, L, iminoglycine, and cationic groups.

As an example of hormonal specificity toward secondary mediators, it may be noted that the effect of thyroid hormones upon amino acid uptake by bone is not mediated by cAMP, whereas that of parathyroid hormone (PTH) is.

It has been suggested that cAMP is identical with the factor in serum which stimulates transport of amino acids into embryonic bone, a role which would classify cAMP with those humoral factors which operate both intra- and extracellularly.

The electrical potential difference across the liver cell membrane is increased by cAMP, cGMP (cyclic guanosine monophosphate), glucagon, and isoproterenol (a synthetic sympathomimetic catecholamine), an effect accompanied by efflux from the cell of Ca^{++} and K^+. Whether these membrane phenomena, which appear to be more rapid than the *in vitro* stimulation of uptake of amino acids by cAMP, have anything to do with the latter remains to be proved.

GLUCAGON. As befits a hormone with general nitrogen-catabolic activity, glucagon facilitates influx of amino acids into liver (where it also promotes catabolism of liver proteins but not of those plasma proteins which are made in the liver). It is not known whether glucagon, as an influence in the hepatotropic direction of nitrogen translocation, has a reciprocal negative effect on amino acid transport in muscle. There is much evidence that the action of glucagon on amino-acid transport, as on amino acid metabolism (to be discussed in later chapters), is mediated by cAMP.

Despite its presumed operation via cAMP, glucagon has no effect *in vivo* on uptake of the L group of amino acids in liver or diaphragm. However, *in vitro* stimulation has been shown for transport into liver of amino acids of the A and cationic groups.

EPINEPHRINE. This hormone, like glucagon, probably functions via cAMP as second messenger. It will be noted in Table 3-1 that epinephrine has opposite effects on transport of amino acids in two groups of tissues and, in fact, on two types of muscle (positive in heart, negative in diaphragm). Injection of epinephrine *in vivo* is reported to facilitate amino acid influx in diaphragm, evidently (since the reverse is seen *in vitro*) by indirect means, such as stimulation of secretion of another hormone (insulin in response to hyperglycemia?).

The catabolically important action of epinephrine in stimulating transport of amino acids into liver can be demonstrated in tissue slices but requires a much longer period of preincubation than glucagon or cAMP. The hepatotropic effect of epinephrine seems to be more potent *in vivo*, suggesting that here, again, at least a part of the final effect of the hormone may be exerted through the mediation of other hormones.

Hormones with Specialized Metabolic Effects

ESTROGENS AND ANDROGENS. Aside from the general protein-anabolic properties of the androgens mentioned earlier, the renotropic effect of androgens, the positive effect of androgens, and the negative effect of estrogens on renal tubular reabsorption of amino acids, most other actions of the gonadal hormones are confined to the reproductive organs and their accessories. The A transport group of amino acids is said to be specifically influenced by estrogens in the uterus.

The actions of the gonadal hormones are slow. Pretreatment of an animal with estrogen for an hour or more and with androgen for many hours is required before an effect can be demonstrated in excised tissues *in vitro*. In the case of estrogen, exposure to the hormone *in vitro* also is successful, but only after prolonged incubation. The evidence suggests that both types of hormones function by stimulating synthesis of one or more proteins involved in the transport mechanism.

PARATHYROID HORMONE.   Uptake of AIB by bone from adult rats is stimulated 8 to 12 hours after administration of PTH but is inhibited by prolonged treatment. Preincubation of embryonic bone with the hormone results in stimulation of uptake of AIB and proline but not leucine (specificity for A system?). cAMP duplicates the action of the hormone in all respects and, hence, is regarded as the mediator.

Uptake of AIB by renal cortical slices is stimulated by PTH, whereas antidiuretic hormone has no effect. These observations are in keeping with the known ability of the former hormone to activate the adenyl cyclase of the renal cortex and the specificity of the latter hormone in stimulating the cyclase in the renal medulla, but not in the cortex.

TROPIC HORMONES.   Although side effects are sometimes observed (e.g., TSH on skeletal muscle and liver), the tropic hormones — adrenocorticotropic, thyrotropic, and follicle-stimulating — exert their influences chiefly upon their appropriate target tissues. cAMP mediates the stimulation of iodide transport in the thyroid gland; the mediation of amino acid transport has not yet been shown to involve cAMP.

Dietary Factors

Liver may adapt to a high-protein diet by augmentation of amino acid transport activity. Increased uptake of AIB has been noted in liver slices taken from rats on such a diet. Glucagon is believed to mediate this adaptation, in turn probably via cAMP.

Skeletal muscle of vitamin E–deficient rabbits takes up AIB at an increased rate, both *in vivo* and *in vitro,* as does the isolated diaphragm. Although the dystrophic muscle caused by this nutritional deficiency in certain animals may exhibit increased permeability to amino acids (and to creatine), the metabolic role of vitamin E in humans is still doubtful, since a nutritional requirement has yet to be demonstrated.

When decreased transport of amino acids was first discovered in animals on vitamin B_6–deficient diets, it was hoped that this finding would lead to the identification of pyridoxine derivatives as prosthetic groups of the transport systems for amino acids, as they are in the case of the transaminases and other enzymes involved in amino-acid metabolism. Unfortunately, the participation of the B_6 group of vitamins in amino acid transport has proved to be quite indirect. One recent explanation of their role has taken note of the deficiency of growth hormone which occurs in this avitaminosis.

Growth and Development

Although even less is known of the factors concerned in regulating the activities of transport systems during growth and development than is known of the analogous factors concerned with enzymes (some of which will be discussed in subsequent chapters), it may be instructive to indicate a few observations showing that transport systems do not remain immutable during the complex biochemical events accompanying growth and differentiation of the organism.

Placental transfer of amino acids to the fetus is reported to be rapid and to have the properties of active transport. Fetal serum contains twice the concentration of amino acids as maternal serum.

Fetal guinea pig liver has low concentrative power toward amino acids, compared to the adult. During the first day after birth this ability rises dramatically in the liver, only slightly in skeletal muscle. After birth, the liver of the rat shows a gradual decrease in amino acid transport activity from initially high toward more adult levels with increasing age.

Developmental studies have contributed to the understanding of the complex problems involving systems for the transport of cystine and the cationic amino acids, discussed in an earlier section. For example, although the uptake of cysteine occurs at adult rates in slices of neonatal rat kidney, that of cystine is markedly deficient and does not reach adult levels until 15 days of age, suggesting two different transport systems developing at different rates. In a similar study, lysine is transported well at an age when cystine is still taken up slowly, again suggesting separate systems.

As has been mentioned earlier, adult kidney contains a common iminoglycine system which transports both glycine and the prolines, as well as more specific systems for transport of the individual amino acids. These conclusions, which are based upon other types of investigations, have been confirmed by developmental studies. Thus, the neonatal rat kidney contains only the common system. With increasing age (1 week) a proline-transporting system emerges, followed in time (3 weeks) by a system specific for glycine as well as that for AIB.

The opposite type of development, namely loss of transport systems with differentiation, has been discussed in connection with the maturation of the erythrocyte. Changes in the same direction are exhibited by the intestinal transport systems for amino acids. Transport of glycine, valine, and lysine by the small intestine of the newborn rat is maximal at 2 to 5 days after birth, after which each of the three systems decreases in activity in a characteristic pattern quite different from the other two.

Qualitative alterations in response to endocrine treatment also appear to be one aspect of the development of transport systems. For example, in the 10-day-old rat, the effect of insulin on AIB uptake by diaphragm is exerted directly upon the membrane carrier mechanism. In the 25-day-old rat, the direct effect is supplemented by an indirect effect which manifests itself in a requirement for protein synthesis related to transport. In the 50-day-old rat, only the indirect effect is seen.

A circadian rhythm is found in the transport of histidine by the rat intestine. The pattern is set by the food intake cycle.

The close relationship between the transport systems for amino acids and those for sugars has been discussed previously. Whatever the basis of this relationship may be, *different* transport systems are involved, as shown by developmental differences between the two groups of systems.

EVALUATION

It may be concluded, on the basis of the observations cited in this chapter, that the major protein-anabolic and protein-catabolic hormones operate in the general directions of mass flow (translocation of nitrogen) discussed in the previous chapter. In those instances in which they do not seem actively to facilitate an expected flux, they at least do not work against it. Nevertheless, it is obvious that the mass flow of nitrogenous metabolites from one tissue to another, in addition to being regulated by alterations in transport systems, also must be controlled by the rates of various intracellular reactions with their attendant changes in size of the metabolic pools of the participants.

In the case of certain specialized tissues, e.g., the reproductive organs, the actions of the regulating hormones seem to make sense. In other tissues, however, outside the major liver-muscle axis, it must be admitted that such regulatory influences as have been reported do not as yet fit into any comprehensive conceptual scheme.

REFERENCES

Characteristics of Transport Systems

Christensen, H. N.: Biological Transport. New York, W. A. Benjamin, Inc., 1962.
Fitch, C.D., Shields, R. P., Payne, W. F., and Dacus, J. M.: Creatine metabolism in skeletal muscle. III. Specificity of the creatine entry process. J. Biol. Chem. *243*:2024–2027 (1968).
Christensen, H. N.: Some special kinetic problems of transport. Adv. Enz. *32*:1–20 (1969).

Characteristics of Individual Tissues

Wilson, T. H.: Intestinal Absorption. Philadelphia, W. B. Saunders Company, 1962, pp. 110–133.
Young, J. A., and Freedman, B. S.: Renal tubular transport of amino acids. Clin. Chem. *17*:245–266 (1971).

Regulation of Amino Acid Transport

Riggs, T. R.: Hormones and the transport of nutrients across cell membranes. *In*: Litwack, G., and Kritchevsky, D. (eds.): Actions of Hormones on Molecular Processes. New York, John Wiley and Sons, Inc., 1964, pp. 1–57.
Riggs, T. R.: Hormones and transport across cell membranes. *In*: Litwack, G., (ed.): Biochemical Actions of Hormones. Vol. 1. New York, Academic Press, Inc., 1970, pp. 157–208.
Koszalka, T. R., and Andrew, C. L.: Effect of insulin on the uptake of creatine-1-^{14}C by skeletal muscle in normal and X-irradiated rats. Proc. Soc. Exptl. Biol. Med. *139*:1265–1271 (1972).

4

DEAMINATION, GLUCONEOGENESIS, AND RELATED PATHWAYS. PART I: DEAMINATION AND CARBON METABOLISM

INTRODUCTION

The preceding chapter has taken amino acids on the first step into the pathways of intermediary metabolism, namely, transport across the cell membrane, whether in the course of intestinal absorption after digestion of proteins or during uptake by the tissues of the body from the extracellular fluids. The pathways available to the amino acids at this point are illustrated in Figure 4-1. Each amino acid in the plasma is in equilibrium with an intracellular pool of the same amino acid, from which pool raw material is taken for both anabolic (e.g., protein synthesis) and catabolic purposes.

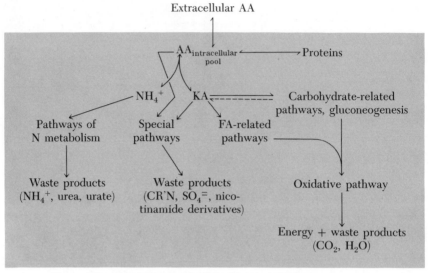

Figure 4–1. Alternative metabolic pathways available to amino acids.

Aside from a few special pathways, the regulation of which will be discussed in a later chapter, the catabolism of most amino acids commences with a deamination, which represents a bifurcation in amino acid metabolism. The nitrogenous branch, beginning with ammonia, will be discussed in the next chapter. This chapter will consider the process of deamination and the subsequent fate of the residual carbon chain, the alpha-keto acid.

The carbon skeletons of most amino acids are readily convertible to precursors of carbohydrate, hence most amino acids can participate in gluconeogenesis, that is, the synthesis of new carbohydrate (i.e., net synthesis) from noncarbohydrate precursors. Most of these glucogenic amino acids are nonessential in the mammalian diet; in a reversal of the aforementioned reactions, carbohydrate can provide the carbon skeletons (alpha-keto acids) of these amino acids, the formation of which is completed by a reversal of the deamination reaction. The keto acid which forms the connecting link between the glucogenic family of amino acids and the carbohydrates is pyruvate (or more properly, phosphoenolpyruvate).

A few amino acids form carbon skeletons which, either with or without glucogenic fragments, yield intermediates which are more closely allied to the fatty acids than to carbohydrate, such as acetate (or acetyl-coenzyme A) or the ketone bodies, acetoacetate, beta-hydroxybutyrate, and acetone. Such fragments cannot participate in net synthesis of carbohydrate. Amino acids which yield such fragments are said to be partly or wholly ketogenic. Since acetate and related carbon skeletons cannot re-form alpha-keto acids, the ketogenic amino acids are not synthesized in the mammal (tyrosine, which might be suggested as an exception to this generalization, is formed only from phenylalanine, another ketogenic amino acid, which is a dietary essential). The compound which provides the connection between the ketogenic amino acids and the pathways of fatty acid metabolism is acetyl-coenzyme A (acetyl-CoA), sometimes simply referred to as acetate.

The pathways of the glucogenic and ketogenic carbon fragments from amino acids converge in acetyl-CoA (readily formed from the glucogenic path by oxidative decarboxylation of pyruvate), which can be oxidized through the Krebs cycle for the production of energy. It is apparent, then, that most of the carbon atoms of amino acids can be channeled into synthesis of carbohydrate (and related compounds), fatty acids (and related compounds), or into a final common pathway of complete oxidation.

GLUCONEOGENESIS AND OTHER GENESES

It has become customary, when discussing the interrelations of amino acids with other metabolites, particularly from the viewpoint of regulatory mechanisms, to confine one's attention to the gluconeogenic pathway and the apparent final goal, the production of blood glucose. There is no doubt that, in conditions of actual or functional carbohydrate deprivation (fasting, diabetes, etc.), the operation of the gluconeogenic pathway is accelerated and that at least a part of this acceleration goes toward a provision of sufficient glucose for the nurture of those tissues which exclusively or at least readily can oxidize glucose for energy purposes, such as the brain. However, these processes and goals are not exclusive. As will be seen later in this chapter, the same conditions which give rise to increased gluconeogenesis from the glucogenic amino acids also cause increased production of acetate and related products from the ketogenic amino acids and, as a matter of fact, also promote lipolysis of fat stores, mobilization of free fatty acids from the adipose depots, increased rates of fatty acid catabolism to ketone bodies (ketogenesis) and acetyl-CoA in the liver, and oxidation of the last through the Krebs cycle.

A more complete picture of the sequelae of carbohydrate deprivation, then, would include not only increased gluconeogenesis (in the sense of actual formation of extra glucose) from amino acids, but also pyruvoneogenesis and acetoneogenesis from amino acids, along with acetoneogenesis from fatty acids, the final goal of these latter processes being ergoneogenesis, or the provision of energy from additional sources.

REGULATION OF THE METABOLISM OF CARBOHYDRATE AND FAT; A BRIEF SUMMARY*

Since, as appears from the preceding arguments, the metabolism of amino acids is interrelated with that of carbohydrates and fats not only by the interchange of raw materials but also by more than merely a coincidence of regulatory mechanisms and predisposing conditions, it is essential at this point to summarize the major factors which control the metabolism of the latter compounds for later comparison with the influences regulating the metabolism of amino acids. This summary is graphically portrayed in Figure 4-2, wherein the pathways of carbohydrate metabolism shown are typical of liver, those of fat metabolism of adipose tissue. With one exception, nonhormonal effectors or modulators of enzyme activity are omitted.

Storage of carbohydrate in the form of glycogen (glycogenesis) is favored by insulin and glucocorticoids. Breakdown of glycogen (glycogenolysis) to form hexose phosphates in liver is accelerated by glucagon and epinephrine (in skeletal muscle only by the latter) and under conditions of fasting and diabetes (some controversy exists on this last point in regard to the human diabetic). As a result of the occurrence of a

---

*More detailed discussions of these pathways and their regulation are to be found in the monographs *Physiological Chemistry of Lipids in Mammals* and *Physiological Chemistry of Carbohydrates in Mammals* of this series, or in a textbook of biochemistry.

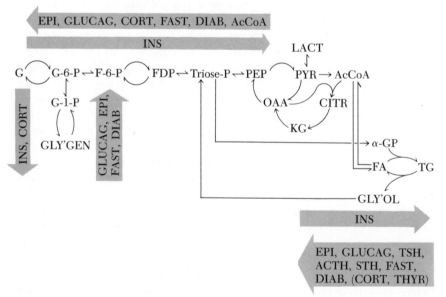

Figure 4–2. Regulation of major metabolic pathways of carbohydrate and fat and their interrelations.

specific phosphatase, accelerated glycogenolysis in liver leads immediately to liberation of glucose into the blood; in muscle the same regulatory influences tend to channel the hexose phosphates into the pathway of glycolysis, with increased formation of lactate.

The major regulatory influence favoring glycolysis, the conversion of glucose or its phosphate esters to the stage of pyruvate-lactate, is insulin. Transformations in the opposite direction, encompassing a large segment of the total process of gluconeogenesis, are stimulated by epinephrine, glucagon, glucocorticoids, and the conditions of fasting and diabetes. In one of several interlocking control mechanisms, acetyl-CoA, a product of fatty acid metabolism, stimulates the gluconeogenic pathway (largely by activating the carboxylation of pyruvate to oxaloacetate). Many other effectors of low molecular weight are reported to influence each of the pathways just discussed; they will not be considered in this monograph.

Although several reactions of the Krebs cycle reportedly are inhibited by free fatty acids or their CoA thioesters *in vitro*, there is considerable doubt concerning the physiological significance of these effects. On the other hand, ATP, the product of the oxidative phosphorylation which accompanies the operation of the Krebs cycle, exerts a restraining influence on the cycle, an example of negative feedback. The close relationship between Krebs cycle components (and pyruvate) and amino acids may be noted: ketoglutarate, oxaloacetate, and pyruvate are directly interconvertible with, respectively, glutamate, aspartate, and alanine, by deamination-reamination reactions. It should also be noted that any amino acid which can furnish a new molecule of pyruvate or a Krebs cycle intermediate can participate in gluconeogenesis; amino acids yielding only acetate type fragments (leucine) are limited to acetoneogenesis and ergoneogenesis.

In adipose tissue a dynamic equilibrium exists between lipogenesis (formation of triglyceride from fatty acids) and lipolysis (the reverse). Reactions in the direction of fat storage are favored by insulin, those in the opposite direction by epinephrine, glucagon, thyrotropic hormone, adrenocorticotropic hormone (effects of the tropic and certain other polypeptide hormones are highly species-specific), growth hormone, and the conditions of fasting and diabetes. Glucocorticoids and thyroid hormones are said to exert a permissive effect in the action of epinephrine. Since lipolysis is accompanied by transport of free fatty acids (attached to plasma albumin) to the extra-adipose tissues such as liver for oxidation, since the resultant increase in acetyl-CoA concentration in the liver cell facilitates gluconeogenesis, and since the glycerol liberated by lipolysis in adipose tissue is not reutilized *in situ* but migrates to other tissues such as liver, where it may contribute raw material for gluconeogenesis, it is evident that, under specific influences, there arises a concerted drive of gluconeogenesis and ergoneogenesis fueled by at least two families of metabolites. Subsequent sections of this chapter will indicate that a third family, the amino acids, also participates. A preview of this has already been seen, insofar as many of the hormonal regulators mentioned here function with regard to amino acids in much the same direction (hepatotropic, etc.) in the phenomena of mass translocation of nitrogen (Chapter 2) and membrane transport (Chapter 3).

FINAL PATHWAYS OF DISPOSAL OF AMINO ACID CARBON
(Fig. 4–3)

Although the carbon skeletons of certain amino acids undergo rather involved metabolic transformations after deamination (and, in some cases, before deamination), most eventually enter into a restricted number of final pathways of disposal, as is illustrated in Figure 4-3.

Those amino acids yielding ketogenic fragments, such as leucine, eventually produce acetyl-CoA or metabolites convertible into it. In the physiological steady-state, fragments of this type may be utilized either for synthesis of fatty acids or oxidized for the production of energy through the Krebs cycle, ignoring, for the sake of simplification, the formation and degradation of ketone bodies. Hormonal or nutritional conditions which lead to the mass transfer of amino acids to the liver for

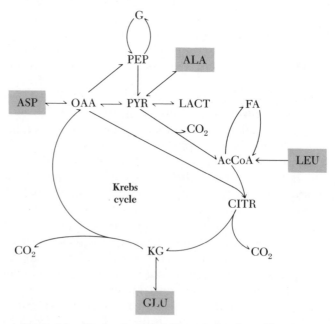

Figure 4–3.   Final pathways of disposal of amino acid carbon.

degradation also are conditions in which synthesis of fatty acids is inhibited; in this case the only pathway available to the acetate fragments is oxidation. The metabolism of amino acid carbon atoms then terminates in CO_2.

Glucogenic amino acids, such as those shown as examples in Figure 4-3 (glutamate, aspartate, alanine), form pyruvate or a member of the Krebs cycle. The pathways of disposal include degradation to CO_2 via the Krebs cycle or formation of carbohydrate (gluconeogenesis in the strict sense). Certain problems arise in the latter case because of the necessity of bypassing irreversible glycolytic reactions as well as the intra- and extramitochondrial localization of certain reactions.

Since the pyruvate kinase step of glycolysis (phosphoenolpyruvate to pyruvate) is not readily reversed, gluconeogenic tissues such as liver and kidney circumvent it by means of a dicarboxylic acid bypass. Pyruvate, if that is the keto acid formed from the glucogenic amino acid in question, is first carboxylated to oxaloacetate by means of pyruvate carboxylase, utilizing the energy of ATP to drive an otherwise endergonic reaction. Oxaloacetate is formed directly from some glucogenic amino acids, indirectly by way of Krebs cycle reactions from others, which initially produce ketoglutarate, succinate, or fumarate. In any case, the next major step in the direction of gluconeogenesis is the conversion of oxaloacetate to phosphoenolpyruvate, catalyzed by phosphoenolpyruvate carboxykinase, with GTP providing the requisite high-energy phosphate group. Subsequent reactions along the pathway to glucose are too far removed from the amino acids to be discussed in this monograph.

In many mammalian species the above-mentioned carboxylase and carboxykinase are localized predominantly in different intracellular compartments, the carboxylation of pyruvate being intramitochondrial, whereas the subsequent formation of phosphoenolpyruvate and the remaining reactions of gluconeogenesis take place in the soluble phase. Since there is general agreement that oxaloacetate is not freely diffusible into or out of the mitochondria, appropriately interconvertible and diffusible substitutes have been sought. Two likely candidates are malate and aspartate. Intramitochondrial oxaloacetate can be reduced to malate by an intramitochondrial malate dehydrogenase or aminated to aspartate by an intramitochondrial glutamate-oxaloacetate transaminase. The malate or aspartate then can diffuse out of the mitochondria into the soluble phase of the cell (cytosol), where oxaloacetate can be regenerated under the influence of extramitochondrial isoenzymes of the particulate enzymes previously mentioned. These mechanisms have been termed *shuttles*.

Thus, fragments from any glucogenic amino acid can circumvent barriers of permeability or of reaction-irreversibility to eventually form glucose.

GENERAL DEAMINATIVE PATHWAYS AND
THEIR REGULATION (Fig. 4-4)

In Figure 4-4, which depicts the major deaminative pathways connected with gluconeogenesis and related metabolic routes, primarily as these occur in liver, it will be noted that the amino acid oxidases are omitted. The feeble and sparsely occurring L-amino acid oxidase has been relegated to the status of a biochemical curiosity for some years. The very active and more widely distributed D-amino acid oxidase, long in limbo on stereochemical grounds, now is accorded a physiological role in mammalian tissues by its probable identity with glycine oxidase. However, neither oxidase plays a significant part in the general pathways now under consideration. There is agreement that the overall process of oxidative deamination of amino acids to keto acids and ammonia (and the reductive amination in the reverse direction) involves two consecutive reactions, as first suggested by Braunstein: transamination of the amino acid in question with ketoglutarate to form glutamate, catalyzed by a specific transaminase, followed by oxidative deamination of glutamate, catalyzed by glutamate dehydrogenase, which is in turn linked with the mitochondrial oxidative chain. The entire process has been termed *transdeamination*.

As can be seen in the figure, glutamate, once formed in the initial transamination, can be reconverted to ketoglutarate by either of two pathways: one, the glutamate dehydrogenase reaction just mentioned, and the other, a transamination with oxaloacetate, catalyzed by glutamate-oxaloacetate transaminase (more recently called aspartate transaminase). The ammonia formed by the dehydrogenase and the aspartate amino group resulting from the transamination contribute the two nitrogen atoms required for urea synthesis via the ornithine cycle. Ammonia is also supplied by the portal blood.

It may be surmised from the figure that regulatory factors could intervene at the following sites: supply of raw material (i.e., the amino acid to be deaminated, AA_X), specific AA_X-transaminase, glutamate dehydrogenase, aspartate transaminase, ornithine cycle, oxidative chain, and Krebs cycle. Regulation of the ornithine cycle will be discussed along with other pathways of disposal of nitrogen (e.g., glutamine synthesis) in the next chapter. There is no evidence that major alterations in the rate of operation of either the oxidative chain or of the Krebs cycle are interrelated with regulation of gluconeogenesis and allied processes, although changes in concentration of certain intermediates of the former pathways (such as ATP, GTP, NAD(P)H, citrate, and acetyl-CoA) may have some influence on the latter; these influences will be mentioned where they apply.

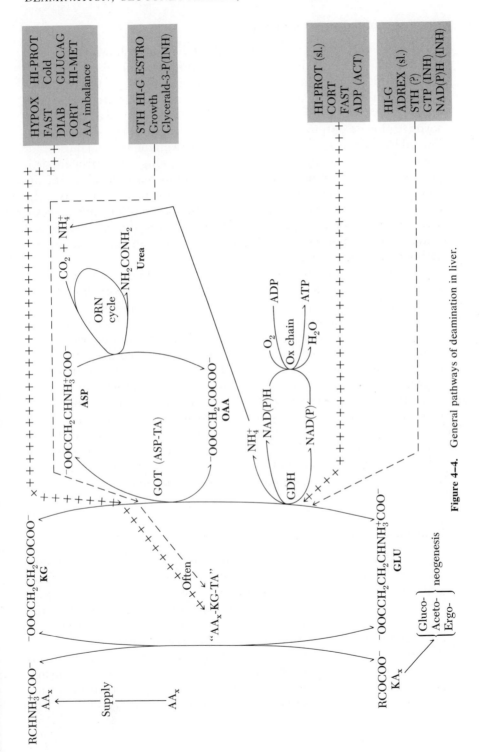

Figure 4-4. General pathways of deamination in liver.

Regulation of Supply of Amino Acid

Recent experiments with perfused rat liver have shown that double the normal plasma amino acid concentration is required even to half-saturate the gluconeogenic mechanism, as measured by the output of glucose and urea. Similarly in man, as determined by differences in arteriovenous concentration in the splanchnic and forearm areas, postabsorptive glucose output by the liver (and to a slight extent, the kidney) is limited by the rate of release of amino acids from the skeletal muscle for uptake by the liver. After several weeks of fasting, gluconeogenesis is greatly reduced in rate, again primarily due to reduced release of peripheral amino acids. (It is of interest that, in these prolonged fasts in the human, kidney becomes a relatively significant site of gluconeogenesis, accounting for some 45 per cent of the total. It is also interesting that alanine is the major amino acid source of glucose, in either the postabsorptive or fasting state.)

If supply is the rate-limiting step in gluconeogenesis from amino acids, then the mechanisms of mobilization and transport discussed in the preceding two chapters are all-important. Consequently, it is legitimate to raise the question, What significance can be attributed to the regulatory mechanisms which are about to be described for the processes of deamination and related pathways? It must be admitted that, at present, no really satisfactory answer is available. One may speculate that most experiments have been performed with the human subject (or the perfused rat liver) in a postabsorptive or fasting state, and that the results may well be different during active absorption of amino acids, or in gluconeogenic states other than fasting, such as high-protein diets and conditions of endocrine imbalance (e.g., diabetes). There is no solid evidence to go on, however, and the situation must simply remain, for now, an embarrassingly rich example of regulatory redundancy.

Regulation of Glutamate Dehydrogenase

Since this enzyme is located within the mitochondria, and since most of the individual amino acid–ketoglutarate transaminases which form glutamate for dehydrogenation are extramitochondrial, it is necessary for glutamate to enter and for ketoglutarate (one of the products of the dehydrogenation) to leave the mitochondria in order to continue the cycle. Both processes of transport have been demonstrated.

Although a very large literature has arisen concerned with the effects of low-molecular-weight modifiers on the activity and conformation of glutamate dehydrogenase, particularly that purified from bovine liver, little is known of its regulation under physiological conditions. The bovine enzyme tends to form more highly aggregated polymers and to exhibit enhanced activity toward glutamate in the presence of adenylates (such as ADP and, under certain conditions, ATP), whereas it usually disaggregates and has less activity toward glutamate in the presence of inhibitors such as GTP, NAD(P)H, certain steroid hormones, and thyroxine. Most, but not all, inhibitors of the bovine enzyme increase its activity as a dehydrogenase of neutral amino acids (such as alanine), although at only a fraction of the activity normally exhibited toward glutamate.

The physiological significance of the above-mentioned effectors is subject to considerable doubt. Many exert their influences only at unphysiologically high concentrations. Others, such as NAD(P)H, ADP, or GTP, which could act as regulators at reasonable intramitochondrial concentrations, do not appear to change sufficiently in concentration with varying rates of gluconeogenesis. Finally, the physiological importance of the aggregation-disaggregation phenomenon in the regulation of glutamate dehydrogenase activity is called into question by the finding that the enzyme from rat liver undergoes no such alterations.

Rat (and frog) liver glutamate dehydrogenase is inactivated by incubation with moderate concentrations of carbamyl phosphate. It is not yet known whether this reaction has any physiological meaning, but, as can be seen in Figure 4-4, it would be useful to the cell to be able to throttle the flow of ammonia from at least one potential source in the face of an accumulation of an intermediate in the major pathway of disposal.

In contrast to the area of activation/inhibition of glutamate dehydrogenase, that of induction/repression appears to offer more evidence of true physiological regulation, although many of the reports in the literature are far from conclusive. Increased levels of the enzyme have been reported to occur in livers of experimental animals on high-protein diets,* during fasting (although there is disagreement in the literature as to the extent and significance of this), and after administration of glucocorticoids, whereas decreases are seen after adrenalectomy and during high-glucose diets. Activity is lower in hypophysectomized animals, probably because of the lack of ACTH. Large doses of growth hormone depress the level further in hypophysectomized rats, but only on *ad libitum* diets.

Although no significant changes have been reported for the diabetic state, it would appear that glutamate dehydrogenase levels otherwise

---

*Although there was no need to mention it previously in connection with the metabolism of carbohydrates or fats, it should be noted that ingestion of a high-protein diet is one of the major conditions causing an increased rate of gluconeogenesis and related processes, since it introduces into the organism a large load of amino acids in the face of limited facilities for storage. Consequently, all avenues of disposal of amino acid nitrogen and carbon are stimulated.

rise and fall with the requirements for gluconeogenesis, granting that the changes have not always been striking, or indeed, reproducible in all instances. Whether the enzyme truly constitutes an important part of the machinery for the transfer of amino acid nitrogen to the ornithine cycle is another question. The equilibrium constant of glutamate dehydrogenase lies far toward the side of amination (of ketoglutarate) and reduction (of NAD or NADP, which are interchangeable *in vitro*, although the latter is said to be preferred in the mitochondrion). Despite a rather high Michaelis constant for NH_3, it is quite possible that the enzyme is not very active in the oxidative direction at those times when NH_3 is plentiful, such as during intestinal absorption, when the portal blood carries rather large amounts of NH_3 to the liver. At such times, of course, the dehydrogenase would not be needed to supply the free NH_3 component of the urea nitrogen. On the other hand, the enzyme represents one of the few sources of free NH_3 in the postabsorptive state.

In the direction of synthesis of nonessential amino acids from keto acids and free NH_3, glutamate dehydrogenase is indispensable. It may be noted that, in addition to accomplishing this synthesis by reversal of the transdeamination pathway, another mechanism is possible. Glutamate dehydrogenase can form a complex with certain transaminases under appropriate experimental conditions. In the presence of ammonia and NADPH, the dehydrogenase converts the transaminase-bound pyridoxal phosphate to bound pyridoxamine phosphate, which then reacts with the appropriate keto acid to form the desired amino acid. The entire complex thus behaves as an amino acid dehydrogenase in reverse.

As for developmental regulation, it may be noted that the process of gluconeogenesis is of no significance during fetal life but becomes increasingly important shortly after birth as a result of the depletion of the store of fetal glycogen and the absence of a maternal supply of blood glucose. Glutamate dehydrogenase belongs to the neonatal developmental group of enzymes (see Chapter 1), which adds some circumstantial evidence for its connection with gluconeogenesis.

Regulation of Aspartate Transaminase

In contrast to glutamate dehydrogenase, aspartate transaminase occurs in liver and other tissues as two distinct isoenzymes, one mitochondrial and the other cytosolic. Although the level of the mitochondrial enzyme is reported to rise and fall under certain conditions and treatments, the soluble isoenzyme appears to be the more responsive in most cases. The following discussion of regulatory factors refers to this cytosolic form of the enzyme unless indicated otherwise.

Since that part of the ornithine cycle which receives its nitrogen in the form of aspartate also is localized in the cytosol, there is no permeability barrier to the interaction of the transaminase with the cycle. Although omitted from Figure 4-4 for simplification, the residual carbon chain of aspartate is actually discharged from the ornithine cycle as fumarate, which is reconverted to oxaloacetate by way of malate in reactions catalyzed by cytoplasmic fumarase and malate dehydrogenase. In this way the aspartate transaminase system acts as a cyclic carrier of half of the nitrogen atoms ultimately found in urea.

As might be anticipated, the level of hepatic cytosolic aspartate transaminase is elevated in typical, gluconeogenic conditions, such as fasting, diabetes, high-protein diets, and administration of glucocorticoids or glucagon, as well as under other circumstances also leading to increased rates of protein catabolism, such as hypophysectomy (loss of growth hormone), cold exposure, imbalanced amino acid diets, and diets containing toxic levels of methionine. In the rat, repeated dosage with glucocorticoid over a period of several days is required to produce an effect and is successful then only in the case of the cytosolic isoenzyme in the male. The effect is blocked by estrogen, which if administered alone lowers the levels of both mitochondrial and cytosolic isoenzymes.

Synthesis of the enzyme appears to be repressed by administration of growth hormone (STH) and, in fact, seems to vary inversely with the growth rate of tissues. A high-glucose diet lowers the level of the mitochondrial isoenzyme, and administration of glucose blocks the induction of the cytosolic isoenzyme by glucocorticoids. The effect of estrogen has been noted in the preceding paragraph.

In addition to these regulatory influences of the induction/repression type, aspartate transaminase activity is inhibited *in vitro* by low concentrations of glyceraldehyde-3-phosphate, which raises the possibility of a rather long-range, negative feedback type of inhibition by a metabolite in the triose stage of glucose synthesis.

Although readily detectable in fetal rat liver, aspartate transaminase exhibits its major developmental spurt from shortly before birth to the first or second postnatal day, then increases somewhat more slowly to about the tenth day, after which it declines gradually to adult values in about a month. Both mitochondrial and cytosolic isoenzymes follow the same pattern.

Injection of glucocorticoids does not affect the development of either isoenzyme until 2 days before birth, at which time the cytosolic isoenzyme alone becomes sensitive to these inducers, a property which it retains at least through the eleventh day after birth. On the other hand, both isoenzymes are induced by thyroxine from 3 to 4 days before birth, but the response is lost by the fourth postnatal day. Estrogen retards development of both isoenzymes.

REGULATION OF DEAMINATION OF INDIVIDUAL AMINO ACIDS AND SUBSEQUENT PATHWAYS OF GLUCONEOGENESIS, ACETONEOGENESIS, AND ERGONEOGENESIS

By way of preface, it should be pointed out that the discussions of pathways of intermediary metabolism of individual amino acids contained within this chapter are restricted to those subsumed under the above title. Pathways leading to the synthesis of special products not involved in the formation of carbohydrate or ketone bodies or in the fairly direct production of energy will be covered in a later chapter.

As was indicated in Figure 4-4, the individual amino acid transaminases often respond to the same regulators and in the same manner as the aspartate transaminase. However, there are sufficient peculiarities among these enzymes as well as among those catalyzing the subsequent reactions of the deaminated carbon skeletons to justify separate treatment. There also exist certain nontransaminative types of deamination which merit individual attention.

The metabolic pathways of the amino acid carbon skeletons can be grouped for purposes of exposition, as shown in Figure 4-5. The grouping is based in part upon sharing a final common metabolite (e.g., pyruvate), in part upon sharing analogous metabolic reactions, even

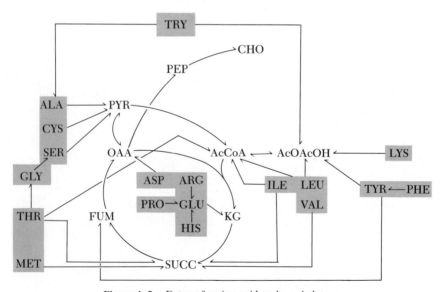

Figure 4–5.   Fates of amino acid carbon skeletons.

though the final products may differ (e.g., the branched-chain amino acids).

The pyruvate family of amino acids, consisting of alanine, cysteine, and serine, are quite directly convertible to this keto acid upon deamination. Glycine will be discussed along with this group because of its intimate metabolic connections with serine. Although the carbon chain of hydroxyproline eventuates in pyruvate, the metabolic pathway of this amino acid parallels that of its parent proline so closely that it will be included with the latter.

Aspartate, glutamate, arginine, histidine, and proline constitute the oxaloacetate-ketoglutarate family of amino acids. The three last-named amino acids are of interest in that they yield ketoglutarate only by first forming another amino acid, glutamate.

Although they differ in many aspects of their metabolism, threonine and methionine share one metabolite (on the pathway to succinate) in common, alpha-ketobutyrate, and are conveniently discussed together.

The branched-chain amino acids undergo almost identical metabolic transformations, and are therefore grouped together, even though leucine is a purely ketogenic amino acid, valine is glucogenic, and isoleucine gives rise to both types of metabolites.

Lysine, tryptophan, and the benzenoid amino acids, phenylalanine and tyrosine, exhibit such individuality in their metabolic pathways that they will be considered separately.

The Pyruvate Family of Amino Acids

ALANINE.   The factors which regulate the hepatic level of alanine transaminase are indicated in Figure 4-6. As in the case of aspartate transaminase, the alanine enzyme occurs as two isoenzymes, one in the mitochondria, one in the cytosol. The figure depicts regulation of the soluble isoenzyme only, since most regulators act similarly on both forms (differences will be noted in the discussion). Also, the ability of all four reactants (alanine, pyruvate, ketoglutarate, and glutamate) to migrate across the mitochondrial membrane makes it a matter of relative indifference, whether alanine enters the mitochondrion for transamination, or undergoes the transformation externally and glutamate enters the particle.

Higher levels of alanine transaminase are induced by diabetes, fasting (no effect reported for mitochondrial isoenzyme), high-protein diet, glucagon, glucocorticoids (effect blocked by administration of glucose or ethionine, an inhibitor of protein synthesis), hypophysectomy, imbalanced amino acid diet or diet containing toxic amounts of methionine (both conditions causing negative nitrogen balance), and exposure to cold. This last-named effect has been shown to be due to increased con-

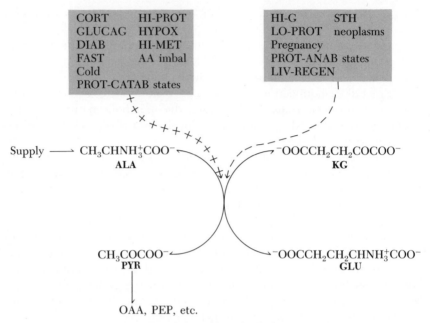

Figure 4–6. Regulation of hepatic alanine transaminase.

sumption of protein, not to the indirect effect of stress and consequent extra secretion of glucocorticoids. In addition to the effects reported after various treatments of the intact animal, glucocorticoid induction of alanine transaminase also has been demonstrated in cultured hepatoma cells.

Lower levels of the enzyme are found on low-protein diets (no change in mitochondrial isoenzyme), high-glucose diets, in livers of rats bearing the Walker carcinoma, in pregnancy, in such protein-anabolic conditions as regenerating liver after partial hepatectomy, and after administration of growth hormone.

In terms of developmental regulation, alanine transaminase differs from glutamate dehydrogenase and aspartate transaminase in that it does not increase significantly in level in rat liver until weaning. However important a role it may play later in life, alanine evidently is not a significant gluconeogenic source in the immediate postnatal period.

Although it exhibits all of the proper responses to regulators which may be expected of an enzyme involved in the process of gluconeogenesis, there is genuine doubt whether alanine transaminase is rate-limiting in this pathway (as discussed earlier in connection with general deamination reactions), and in fact, when alterations in its level are observed, whether these represent cause or effect. The first doubt is occasioned by the observation that, in certain experimental situations, the rate of gluconeogenesis is limited by the *supply* of amino acids (especially alanine) transported to the liver, suggesting that the effects of various regulatory factors in peripheral tissues are more significant than whatever they may do to enzymes in the liver. The question of cause and effect is raised by experiments in which the actual rate of induction of alanine transaminase in rat liver is compared with the rate of synthesis of glycogen after administration of glucocorticoid hormone. Glycogen deposition begins within 2 hours; the transaminase does not begin to increase in level until after a lag of 2 to 12 hours. Hence, this enzyme and other slowly induced enzymes in this pathway may not be causative agents in the increased rate of gluconeogenesis, but rather may be examples of adaptation of the cell to handle current and possible future increased fluxes of material, with the increase more directly referable to some other truly rate-limiting step.

Whatever the significance of hepatic regulation, there is no doubt of the importance of alanine as source material for gluconeogenesis, as mentioned in earlier sections of this chapter. Indeed, an alanine cycle has been postulated (by analogy with the Cori cycle), in which alanine transports amino acid nitrogen from muscle to liver, where, after deamination, the carbon skeleton forms glucose which is returned to muscle. There, glycolysis results in the production of pyruvate, from which alanine can be re-formed, thus completing the cycle. Alanine also may function as a negative allosteric effector of pyruvate kinase, and by so doing may decrease the rate of glycolysis relative to that of gluconeogenesis.

After deamination, the carbon skeleton of alanine, in the form of the keto acid, pyruvate, enters the route to carbohydrate synthesis by carboxylation to oxaloacetate, as previously described. Depending upon physiological requirements, pyruvate alternatively may be decarboxylated oxidatively to acetyl-CoA, the possible disposal of which also has been discussed.

CYSTEINE. Figure 4-7 outlines the major reactions involved in the catabolism of cysteine. It will be noted that the reactions connecting the metabolism of methionine with that of cysteine are indicated only briefly, despite the very close interrelationship of these two amino acids from the standpoint of sulfur metabolism. The coupling of the discussion of methionine metabolism with that of threonine rather than cysteine in this monograph is based upon a consideration of the fate of the deaminated carbon chains; methionine may donate its sulfur to the biosynthesis of cysteine, but its carbon chain is more closely allied with that derived from threonine, whereas the cysteine carbon chain is provided by serine.

There seems little doubt that cysteine (and cystine, its oxidation product with which it is readily interconvertible) should be classified as a glucogenic amino acid, as may be seen from the five possible pathways to pyruvate indicated in Figure 4-7. The occasional lack of success in demonstrating glucogenicity reported in the older literature may perhaps be attributed to the contribution of nonglucogenic pathways, and to the rather devious character of the truly glucogenic pathways. The latter must include, in addition to a deamination step, some provision for removal of sulfur; it is quite possible that one or more of the intermediary reactions is rather slow.

The catabolic pathways of cysteine are irreversible, in the practical, overall sense. Since cysteine is nonessential, it must be synthesized in the animal organism, which it is, but by pathways different from the catabolic. Carbohydrate furnishes the carbon chain by way of serine, whereas the sulfur, as mentioned previously, is provided by the essential amino acid methionine.

As will be noted in Figure 4-7, there exist in mammalian liver both intra- and extramitochondrial reactions which participate in the catabolism of cysteine. One mitochondrial pathway leads to the formation of pyruvate, sulfate, and glutamate. Unfortunately, little is known of the intermediary reactions. It has been hypothesized that cysteine may be deaminated initially to beta-mercaptopyruvate, probably by transamination with ketoglutarate (a reaction of this type is known to take place in the cytosol), followed by cleavage of the sulfur, either before or after oxidation, with the eventual appearance of the sulfur as sulfate and the carbon chain as pyruvate.

A second pathway leading to mitochondrial formation of pyruvate actually begins in the cytosol. Cysteine is oxidized by a soluble oxygenase to cysteine sulfinate which, among other alternatives, may enter the mitochondria. There it is oxidatively deaminated by an NAD-linked dehydrogenase to form the unstable beta-sulfinylpyruvate, which decomposes to pyruvate and hyposulfite, the latter being oxidized further to sulfate.

Cysteine oxygenase is induced in intact rats by both glucocorticoids and cysteine, but in adrenalectomized animals only by the former when each is used singly. These observations suggest that substrate induction does not exist as such in this system but depends upon adrenal intervention. However, administration of cysteine along with glucocorticoid in adrenalectomized rats results in considerable enhancement of the degree of induction over that produced by the hormone alone. Thus, it is possible that substrate induction can occur in the presence of permissive quantities of adrenal hormone. As will be noted later, an analogous situation exists in the case of tyrosine transaminase.

Another pathway for the conversion of cysteine sulfinate to pyruvate occurs in the cytosol. In this case, the deamination is catalyzed by a transaminase utilizing ketoglutarate. The remaining reactions resemble those described in the preceding paragraph.

Cysteine also can be deaminated in the cytosol by a transaminase

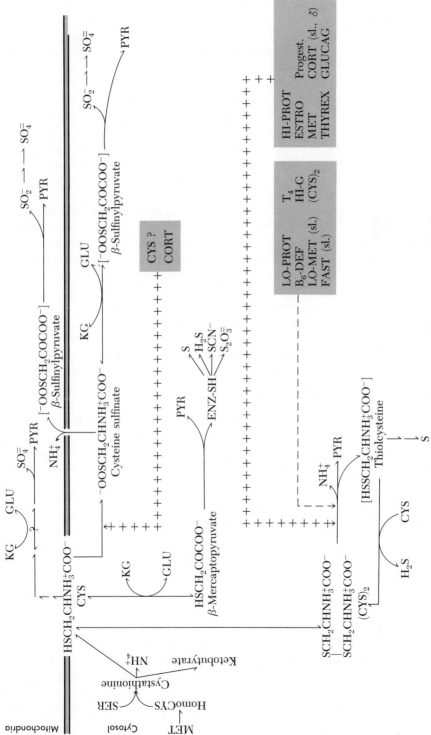

Figure 4–7. Pathways of cysteine catabolism in mammalian liver.

system which has not been well characterized, yielding beta-mercap-topyruvate (thiolpyruvate), which is attacked by a thiolpyruvate-cleaving enzyme, producing pyruvate and enzyme-bound thiol. The latter may decompose to elemental sulfur or may react with reducing substances in the cell to yield H_2S, with traces of cyanide to yield thiocyanate, or with sulfite to yield thiosulfate.

The final pathway to be considered used to be called the cysteine desulfhydrase route, supposedly catalyzed by an enzyme which, by anal-ogy with the serine-threonine dehydratase (see later sections of this chapter), removes from the amino acid the elements of H_2S (instead of H_2O), producing an unstable intermediate which would decompose to ammonia and pyruvate. It is now realized that both enzyme and sub-strate were incorrectly identified.

The reaction which produces NH_3, H_2S, and pyruvate in the cytosol is catalyzed by cystathionase, the same enzyme which cleaves cystathio-nine in the pathway from methionine to cysteine (to be discussed under methionine). Pyridoxal phosphate is the coenzyme. The substrate is cys-tine, the oxidized derivative of cysteine. In the enzyme reaction proper, ammonia and pyruvate are produced, along with the unstable thiolcys-teine, which may decompose to release elemental sulfur, or may react with cysteine in the cell to release H_2S and regenerate cystine.

The level of this desulfhydrase reaction (or of the cystathionase re-action) in liver is increased by a high-protein diet, administration of es-trogen, progesterone, glucocorticoids (slightly and in male rats only), methionine, glucagon, and thyroidectomy. The level is decreased by a low-protein or high-glucose or low-methionine (small effect) diet, fasting (slightly), thyroid hormones, and pyridoxine deficiency. Both repression and inhibition of the enzyme by cystine have been reported. Aside from several idiosyncrasies, such a pattern of regulation would be expected from a reaction important in gluconeogenesis. Unfortunately, little or nothing is known of the regulation of several of the other reaction sequences leading from cysteine to pyruvate, so that no estimate of rela-tive glucogenic potential can be made at this time. It must also be kept in mind that the cystathionase reaction responds to the same regulatory in-fluences; in certain cases the regulator seems to be more appropriate to cystathionase than to desulfhydrase, e.g., repression or inhibition by cys-tine, which makes sense as an example of negative feedback by me-tabolite in the case of cystathionase (which produces cysteine and therefore cystine), but makes no sense for the desulfhydrase reaction, for which cystine is the substrate. The cystathionase reaction will be dis-cussed in greater detail under methionine metabolism.

Perhaps a comment is called for at this point in connection with the interrelation of thyroid hormones and pyridoxine derivatives. Over the years, it has been noted that the activity of certain enzymes requiring pyridoxal phosphate as coenzyme is depressed after administration of thyroid hormones and elevated by thyroidectomy. In some cases, it has been demonstrated that thyroid hormones (in excess) produce a deficiency of vitamin B_6 (pyridoxine) and its derivatives in the tissues with concomitant loss of activity of those enzymes dependent upon the related cofactors. Activity is restored by *in vivo* administration of the vitamin or *in vitro* addition of pyridoxal phosphate to the enzyme assay system. Consequently, the generalization has sometimes appeared in the older literature that thyroid hormones exert their influence on enzyme activity solely through the vitamin, as indicated. However, the generalization is not valid. Although thyroid hormones certainly can affect the tissue level of pyridoxine derivatives, they can also raise or lower the level of apoenzymes quite independently of their cofactors. Conversely, pyridoxine can raise the level of enzyme activity by true induction of *de novo* protein synthesis. Thus, it is necessary to examine each individual case before drawing conclusions.

SERINE. Figure 4-8 outlines the major anabolic and catabolic pathways of serine metabolism and the known regulatory influences. Two pathways will be rather summarily dismissed at this point, not on the grounds of lack of importance, but because they are more appropriately discussed elsewhere. A certain amount of serine must be disposed of daily through condensation with a homocysteine residue from methionine to form cystathionine and, eventually, cysteine. This pathway will be deferred until the metabolism of methionine is taken up, since there is no evidence that it is a major route of gluconeogenesis from serine. Likewise, the serine-glycine interconversion reaction, although it forms the probable chief source of carbohydrate-derived raw material for synthesis of glycine when needed, is mainly of importance as a catabolic route for glycine in conditions of gluconeogenesis, and hence will be discussed in connection with glycine in the next section.

This section will begin with a consideration of the biosynthetic pathways to serine, first, because they illustrate the close connection of that amino acid to carbohydrate and second, because these routes, running in the opposite sense, at times have been suggested as possible pathways in gluconeogenesis from serine.

To start with, it should be noted that two of the compounds in Figure 4-8 are in the mainstream of glycolysis, namely 2- and 3-phosphoglycerate. Hexose and triose phosphates readily form 3-phosphoglycerate, which in turn initiates the so-called phosphorylated biosynthetic pathway to serine. The first enzyme in this pathway, 3-phosphoglycerate dehydrogenase, produces phosphohydroxypyruvate, which is in turn acted upon by phosphohydroxypyruvate transaminase to form phosphoserine. A specific phosphatase, the only really irreversible enzyme in the series, hydrolyzes phosphoserine to serine. It is doubtful whether serine can be phosphorylated directly in the free state; no kinase catalyzing such a reaction has been reported. However,

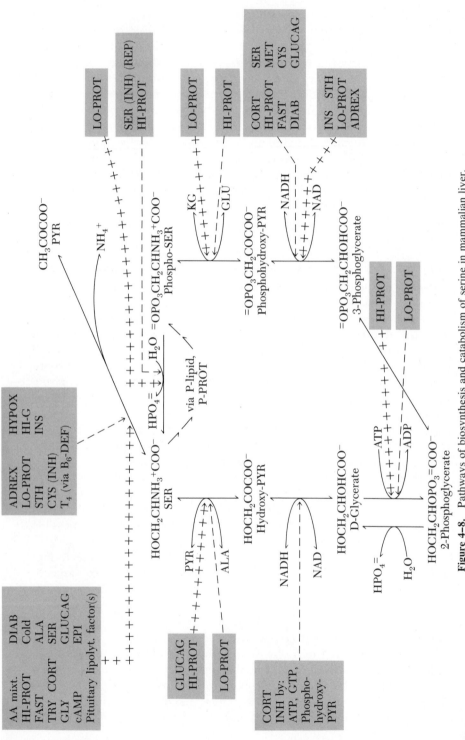

Figure 4–8. Pathways of biosynthesis and catabolism of serine in mammalian liver.

phosphoserine residues in bound form appear in certain phospholipids and phosphoproteins. If the phosphoserine of these sources were available for general metabolism, then the entire phosphorylated pathway would be physiologically reversible.

In parallel with the above, there also exists a nonphosphorylated biosynthetic pathway. 2-Phosphoglycerate can be hydrolyzed by a specific phosphatase to yield D-glycerate (also possibly derived from fructose-1-phosphate by means of an aldolase which forms dihydroxyacetone phosphate and D-glyceraldehyde, followed by oxidation of the latter). D-Glycerate dehydrogenase forms hydroxypyruvate, which transaminates with alanine to yield pyruvate and serine. The entire sequence is made physiologically reversible by the existence of a kinase which permits re-phosphorylation of D-glycerate.

A pathway for the biosynthesis of a nonessential amino acid from carbohydrate should have certain characteristics, such as high levels of activity during periods of rapid growth and in other protein-anabolic situations, and conversely, lower levels of activity in conditions of accelerated protein catabolism, particularly during enhanced gluconeogenesis. The phosphorylated biosynthetic pathway to serine fits these requirements rather well.

3-Phosphoglycerate dehydrogenase, the first and probably rate-limiting enzyme in the phosphorylated pathway, is found in increased concentration in liver of animals on low-protein diets, conditions under which an increased requirement for serine biosynthesis would be anticipated. The rise is prevented by inclusion of extra cysteine or methionine in the diet. Increased concentration of the dehydrogenase is found also after adrenalectomy, or administration of insulin or growth hormone. Decreased hepatic levels of this enzyme occur in experimental animals on high-protein diets, in fasting, in diabetes, and after administration of glucocorticoids or glucagon. The rate of synthesis of serine by human cells in culture is diminished by the presence of preformed serine, in part due to repression of synthesis of the dehydrogenase (actions on the phosphatase in this sequence will be discussed shortly).

Phosphohydroxypyruvate transaminase activity in liver, as in the case of the preceding enzyme, bears a roughly reciprocal relationship to the level of protein in the diet.

Phosphoserine phosphatase levels also vary inversely with the concentration of protein in the diet, and, in cell culture, are repressed by the presence of serine. In addition, the phosphatase in inhibited strongly by serine in the usual range of tissue concentrations of this amino acid, providing another example of product (or metabolite) repression of enzyme synthesis together with inhibition of enzyme activity.

In consonance with the regulatory properties of a biosynthetic rather than gluconeogenic pathway, the dehydrogenase and phosphatase of the phosphorylated pathway both have been found to arise in the late fetal rather than neonatal period of development.

The role of the nonphosphorylated pathway, unfortunately, is not nearly as clear. Most investigators agree that the phosphorylated pathway predominates in fetal life. In the adult there appears to be great species variation with respect to the relative importance of the two pathways. Furthermore, it is not at all certain whether the nonphosphorylated route is biosynthetic or catabolic. For example, the serine-pyruvate transaminase and D-glycerate kinase levels are both increased on high-protein and decreased on low-protein diets, the transaminase is induced by administration of glucagon, and the transaminase as well as the D-glycerate dehydrogenase both develop during the neonatal period, all properties consistent with a gluconeogenic function. Bovine liver D-glycerate dehydrogenase activity is inhibited by a number of nucleotides, of which ATP and GTP are the most potent. Such a phenomenon would be a useful regulatory mechanism in an ergogenic path. The enzyme is inhibited also by a member of the phosphorylated pathway, phosphohydroxypyruvate, perhaps as a means of retarding a catabolic pathway while a parallel anabolic route is in full operation. On the other hand, the dehydrogenase is repressed by administration of glucocorticoids, which is certainly aberrant from this point of view.

In contrast to the preceding, there is little doubt that the serine dehydratase reaction represents the major catabolic pathway for serine, and the chief gluconeogenic route for serine and probably for glycine as well. It should be mentioned before going on that in most mammalian species serine dehydratase and threonine dehydratase are one and the same enzyme, an identity which should be kept in mind when regulation is discussed. On the other hand, the previously presumed identity of this enzyme with cystathionine synth(et)ase has been shown to be erroneous.

Hepatic levels of serine dehydratase are increased by a high-protein diet, administration of amino acid mixtures or certain individual amino acids (serine, glycine, alanine, tryptophan) under specific experimental conditions, glucocorticoids, fasting, diabetes, exposure to cold, a pituitary lipolytic fraction, cAMP, and hormones probably mediated by this nucleotide (glucagon, epinephrine). Of great interest are recent reports to the effect that, of two electrophoretically separable isoenzymes of the dehydratase having the same molecular weight, the more electropositive (type I) is induced specifically by glucocorticoids, the more electronegative (type II) by glucagon. Type II predominates in intact rats on standard laboratory chow, the diabetic, the newborn, and in adrenalectomized rats on relatively low-protein diets. High-protein diets or protein-free diets supplemented with tryptophan produce roughly equal amounts of the two forms in intact rats, probably through supplementary adrenal cortical stimulation of production of type I, along with type II.

Comparison of the specific activity of serine dehydratase in the livers of several species of mammals of widely different size (from the shrew to the sheep) yields an inverse relationship with size (similar to the well-known relationship of size and basal metabolic rate).

Cysteine inhibits serine dehydratase *in vitro*. Lowered levels of the enzyme are seen after adrenalectomy, hypophysectomy, low-protein diets, and administration of growth hormone or insulin. Although thyroid hormones have been reported in the past to induce the enzyme, more recent investigations have shown decreased specific activity (due to diminished tissue concentration of pyridoxal phosphate) as well as less apoenzyme (presumed to be caused by increased lability in the absence of cofactor). Glucose represses the basal rate of synthesis of the dehydratase, as well as antagonizing the inductive effect of certain other agents. This glucose effect, which resembles an analogous phenomenon of widespread occurrence in microorganisms, is believed to be independent of insulin action, to take place probably at the level of translation, and to function possibly by blocking release of polyribosome-bound enzyme.

In keeping with its function as a gluconeogenic enzyme, serine dehydratase exhibits its first developmental spurt in the rat during the neonatal period. A steeper rise in activity is seen around weaning, after which the level falls off to adult values at about 1 month of age. Synthesis of the enzyme can be evoked prematurely by glucagon administration to the rat fetus, an induction which is repressible by insulin.

Despite the generally consistent picture presented in the foregoing paragraphs, a few doubts have been raised by recent reports from one laboratory. It is pointed out that serine dehydratase has a rather high Michaelis constant for serine, possibly too high for efficient physiological action. Also, in the perfused liver, glucose formation from serine is claimed not to be inhibited by quinolinate, a tryptophan metabolite which specifically inhibits phosphoenolpyruvate carboxykinase, a key enzyme on the presumed route from serine through pyruvate to glucose. Finally, the pattern of isotope labeling resulting from labeled serine is said to be inconsistent with pyruvate as an intermediate. The phosphorylated or nonphosphorylated biosynthetic routes are suggested as possible alternatives. It must be noted that disagreement with these reports has already been registered from another laboratory.

GLYCINE. As can be seen in Figure 4-9, glycine metabolism appears to be characterized by a plethora of metabolic routes combined with a dearth of regulatory information. Several pathways not primarily concerned with either biogenesis or degradation of glycine are omitted from the figure: formation of creatine, glutathione, porphyrins, or purines and various conjugation reactions, such as synthesis of glycocholates, hippurates, etc.

It is generally accepted at this time that glycine is glucogenic. Although this view was held by early investigators, largely on the basis of balance experiments on diabetic animals, later workers were unable to obtain consistent results, and several concluded that glycine stimulated

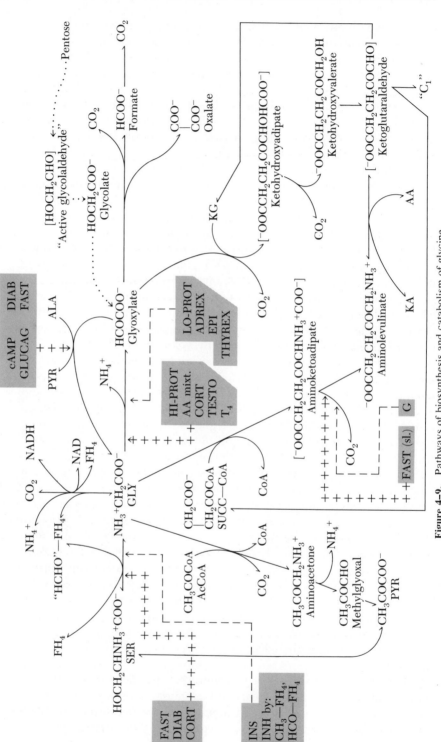

Figure 4-9. Pathways of biosynthesis and catabolism of glycine.

the formation of carbohydrate rather than contributing to it directly. On the basis of isotopic tracer experiments, it seems clear that glycine is convertible to glucose. However, the route of conversion is indirect (probably proceeding through the intermediate formation of serine) and may be slow.

Several reports in the literature discuss the regulation of glycine synthesis and degradation in terms of the overall processes; although these findings do not specify individual metabolic reactions, they are nevertheless useful in construction of a general framework of ideas into which finer details can be fitted later. Thus, glycine is reported to repress its own biosynthesis in cell culture. On the catabolic side, the overall rate of conversion of glycine to ammonia is increased on a high-protein diet. The incorporation of labeled glycine carbon into glucose is increased by glucocorticoids, decreased by insulin and by glucose. It should be noted that, since a large part of glycine metabolism may well proceed through serine, the regulatory influences just mentioned could be exerting their effects through the latter amino acid.

The pathway of glycine catabolism which can be considered classic, largely on the basis of seniority, is its aerobic oxidative deamination to glyoxylate. This reaction was formerly attributed to the action of a specific glycine oxidase, but comparative studies over the years now make it seem probable that glycine oxidase is identical with D-amino acid oxidase. Recent findings with respect to other pathways may perhaps diminish the significance formerly accorded the oxidase in glycine catabolism; nevertheless, a summary of known regulatory influences may be of interest. (No attempt is made in the following to differentiate glycine oxidase from D-amino acid oxidase, in view of their probable identity.)

Hepatic levels of the oxidase are higher on high-protein diets or after administration of amino acid mixtures, glucocorticoids, thyroid hormones, or androgens. Growth hormone has no effect. Lower levels are seen on low-protein diets, administration of epinephrine, or after thyroidectomy or adrenalectomy. Studies after hypophysectomy have been contradictory, and some of the results with androgens have been inconsistent. Developmentally, the liver enzyme increases in activity postnatally but does not approach adult levels until weaning. As can be seen, although the oxidase exhibits a few of the attributes of the gluconeogenic enzymes, most of its characteristics are individual. Actually, there appears to be no way in which this enzyme could be involved in gluconeogenesis, since glyoxylate is not glucogenic.

The further oxidation of glyoxylate proceeds through formation of CO_2 and formate, which in turn is oxidized to CO_2. If glyoxylate accumulates in higher than usual concentrations, it is oxidized to oxalate, which is not metabolized further. No regulatory mechanisms have been reported for these reactions.

Several transaminases have been discovered which catalyze irreversible conversions of glyoxylate to glycine. One of these, an alanine-glycine transaminase, since it is induced in liver by glucagon, cAMP, diabetes, and fasting, has been proposed as the first enzyme in a gluconeogenic sequence leading from glyoxylate through glycine and serine. As already mentioned, glyoxylate is not demonstrably glucogenic, and glycine is evidently not strongly so. However, such a pathway, albeit feeble, may exist; as will be noted shortly, the glycine-serine interconversion step is subject to typical gluconeogenic regulatory influences. A more serious obstacle to the proposal concerns the source of glyoxylate. Its possible origin in glycolate, which in turn could derive from the active glycolaldehyde involved in pentose metabolism, leads to the rationally unsatisfactory and metabolically wasteful situation of glucogenic raw material orginating in carbohydrate. Unhappily, no other major source of glyoxylate is known at this time. (A minor source is hydroxyproline.)

Further study of the aforementioned transaminase has revealed the existence of both mitochondrial and cytosolic isoenzymes. The increased enzyme level in rat liver after administration of glucagon is due entirely to the particulate enzyme, which also is believed to be the isoenzyme more directly involved in gluconeogenesis. In the rat, the mitochondrial isoenzyme begins to develop in the late fetal liver, increases from birth to a peak above adult levels in 10 days, and then decreases to normal adult levels. The cytosolic isoenzyme begins to develop prenatally, increases after birth to a plateau at 6 days, and then at about 15 days rises to adult levels. Premature induction of the mitochondrial isoenzyme occurs after administration of thyroxine, glucagon, or cAMP, the response to glucagon disappearing by the second postnatal day. The cytosolic isoenzyme may be induced prematurely by thyroxine or glucocorticoid; the latter response remains until the fifth postnatal day and may be evoked even on the twelfth day if coupled with casein intubation.

Three routes of glycine catabolism which are considered of minor quantitative significance are the succinate-glycine cycle, the carboligase cycle, and the aminoacetone pathway. In the first of these, which actually comprises the first part of the biosynthetic route to the porphyrins, glycine and succinyl-CoA condense to form a labile intermediate which loses CO_2, producing aminolevulinate. The synth(et)ase which catalyzes this reaction is repressed by glucose and induced moderately by fasting, but its major regulatory aspects will be discussed in connection with the synthesis of porphyrins, in which it plays a much more important role. Aminolevulinate can be transaminated to the labile ketoglutaraldehyde, which may lose a one-carbon fragment of the formate or formaldehyde type and become succinate, or may be oxidized to ketoglutarate, which can form succinate (or succinyl-CoA) by oxidative decarboxylation, thus completing the cycle in either case.

In the carboligase cycle, glyoxylate condenses with ketoglutarate to form a labile intermediate which loses CO_2, producing ketohydroxy-valerate, which by oxidation forms ketoglutaraldehyde, the reactions of which are the same as in the previously discussed pathway. It should be noted that both of these pathways result in complete degradation of the carbon chain of glycine to CO_2 or one-carbon fragments. Neither route could be used for gluconeogenesis or related processes.

The third pathway begins with the condensation of glycine and acetyl-CoA to form aminoacetone (also derivable from threonine), which is oxidized by an amine oxidase to methylglyoxal. Through the operation of the so-called glyoxylase system, or more directly (as shown in the figure) by the action of a dehydrogenase, pyruvate is produced, hence this pathway is potentially gluconeogenic. Regulatory studies have not been reported for the carboligase or aminoacetone pathways.

One of the major reactions of glycine metabolism is its interconversion with serine, catalyzed by an enzyme variously called (in accord with its demonstrated specificity) serine transhydroxymethylase, serine hydroxymethylase, serine aldolase, or threonine aldolase. Its role in threonine metabolism will be discussed in a later section. Although pyridoxal phosphate is a coenzyme for the reaction, tetrahydrofolate serves as carrier of the one-carbon (hydroxymethyl) unit, on the oxidation level of formaldehyde, which is reversibly added to glycine to form serine.

The transhydroxymethylase level of the uterus is increased by administration of estrogen, and that of the jejunum, not usually considered a target of gonadal hormones, is increased by androgen in the male and estrogen in the female. Jejunal enzyme also is reported to be higher on a folate-containing than folate-free diet, and to be highest on a high-carbohydrate diet, next highest on a high-protein diet, and lowest in fasting. A possible indication that the glycine-serine conversion represents a step in a gluconeogenic sequence is provided by unpublished results tabulated in a review article, to the effect that hepatic transhydroxymethylase levels are increased by glucocorticoids, fasting, and diabetes and are decreased by insulin. The importance of the beta carbon atom of serine as a source of one-carbon units is pointed up by the inhibition of the activity of this enzyme by methyl-tetrahydrofolate and formyl-tetrahydrofolate, an example of metabolite negative feedback.

The most recently discovered metabolic pathway of glycine is the cleavage reaction, in which glycine is reversibly split into ammonia, CO_2, and a formaldehyde fragment carried by tetrahydrofolate. Since a molecule of glycine, via this reaction, can provide the one-carbon unit required by the transhydroxymethylase to convert glycine to serine, a combined reaction can be set up, utilizing the two processes, in which two molecules of glycine are utilized to synthesize one molecule of serine. Although regulatory properties of the cleavage system have not been reported, it is quite possible that the combined reactions serve to synthesize glycine under ordinary circumstances but operate in the direction of serine formation from glycine when the metabolic signals call for gluconeogenesis.

The Oxaloacetate-Ketoglutarate Family of Amino Acids

Glutamate and Aspartate. The function of these two amino acids as catalytic carriers of nitrogen in the general process of deamination has been depicted in Figure 4-4 and discussed in the accompanying text. When present in greater than required concentrations, both amino acids lose nitrogen in the usual manner, then contribute their carbon skeletons, in the forms of ketoglutarate and oxaloacetate, to the gluconeogenic pathway. The routes were outlined in Figure 4-3 and involve conversion to phosphoenolpyruvate, either directly or after traversing part of the Krebs cycle. Regulatory mechanisms are the same as those involved in the catalytic functions of glutamate and aspartate.

It should be noted that, since the remaining members of this metabolic family (arginine, histidine, and proline) enter the gluconeogenic pathway only after prior conversion to glutamate, they are each subject to whatever regulatory influences affect the catabolism of glutamate, in addition to those controls which may function in their several metabolic routes up to the common intermediate.

Arginine (Fig. 4-10). A major difficulty in attempting to discuss the metabolism of arginine is posed by the impossibility of separating those reactions assignable strictly to the chief routes of biosynthesis and catabolism of arginine from reactions related to the function of arginine and allied compounds as members of the ornithine cycle (see Chapter 5). Part of the problem derives from the fact that several of the reactions of the ornithine cycle not only participate in the chiefly catabolic function of that cycle but also operate in an anabolic sense, subserving the synthesis of important products. Reactions (or cycles) having such dual functions are said to be *amphibolic*. Other reactions of arginine and its derivatives, outside the ornithine cycle proper, although having independent functions, also may be sources of cycle intermediates, replenishing these when required. By analogy with the Krebs cycle, where such a term was first applied, these refilling reactions may be called *anaplerotic*.

As shown in Figure 4-10, the two reactions of interest in this section are the conversion of arginine to urea and ornithine (catalyzed by arginase), and deamination of the latter to glutamate semialdehyde (catalyzed by ornithine delta-transaminase). The semialdehyde may be reversibly converted to glutamate or, in two steps, to proline (to be discussed in a later section).

Before discussing regulation, it may be instructive to outline briefly the possible metabolic roles of the reactions at hand. For example, in the operations of the ornithine cycle as a catabolic disposal mechanism for

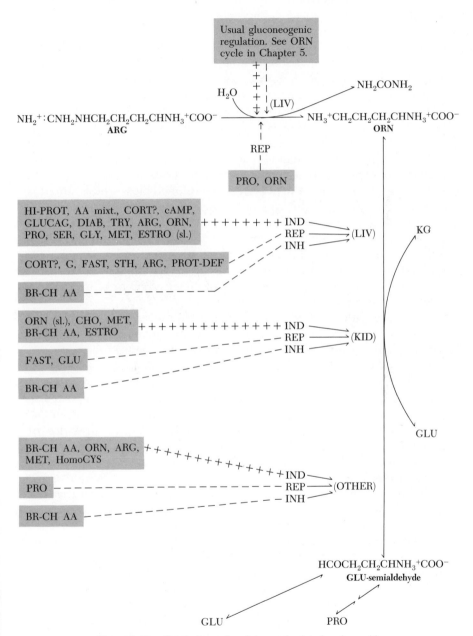

Figure 4–10. Catabolism of arginine and related amino acids.

ammonia, arginase plays a catalytic role, whereas ornithine transaminase may be acting anaplerotically. In the process of gluconeogenesis from arginine (and ornithine), a net degradation of these two raw materials to glutamate, ketoglutarate, etc., is required, whereas this same process of gluconeogenesis calls for increased activity of the ornithine cycle and hence increased concentrations of cycle intermediates, thus giving rise to apparently contradictory metabolic signals. In the biosynthesis of arginine from carbohydrate intermediates, ornithine transaminase and most of the reactions of the ornithine cycle function anabolically. In proline biosynthesis, if carbohydrate is the immediate raw material, then the reactions of ornithine and arginine can be bypassed, since the route need utilize only glutamate semialdehyde; however, if arginine is the source, then this biosynthesis requires that ornithine transaminase operate in a sense opposite to that of the previously mentioned biosynthesis, and it is also of interest that, in this case, arginase plays an anabolic role.

In addition to the above considerations, further complications are caused by the occurrence of several reactions of arginine and ornithine (but not the entire ornithine cycle) in extrahepatic tissues, notably kidney. Whatever the functions of the various reactions may be in these sites, synthesis of urea is not one of them. (Small amounts of urea *can* be synthesized in brain.)

The regulation of liver arginase will be dismissed briefly in this section, since it is necessary to consider it in greater detail in connection with the ornithine cycle in Chapter 5. It will suffice at this point to state, as indicated in Figure 4-10, that liver arginase is subject to the usual factors which are encountered whenever regulated reactions play roles in the gluconeogenic pathway. In addition, arginase levels are reported to be repressed in cultured liver cells by the presence of proline or ornithine (metabolite repression) and are induced by the presence of arginine in other cells (HeLa). Ornithine (and its analog, lysine) acts as a competitive inhibitor of arginase generally. These various effects may be related to the conversion of arginine to proline in liver, although, as will be seen in Chapter 5, arginase is present in such excess in liver that it is doubtful whether any reasonable increase or decrease in its level can alter the course of metabolic pathways.

Kidney arginase appears to be largely uninfluenced by many of the factors which affect the liver enzyme. Conversely, certain regulators appear to be directed at the kidney enzyme, with little or no effect in the liver. For instance, kidney arginase is not influenced by the level of protein, but is induced by addition of proline to the diet. Testosterone increases the arginase level in the kidneys of mature male rats and immature rats of both sexes, but in mature females only after ovariectomy. The significance of these observations with respect to arginine metabolism in the kidney is obscure at present.

In contrast to arginase, which is soluble, ornithine transaminase is mitochondrial in location, which places it (in liver, at least) in advantageous proximity to the enzyme which draws ornithine into the cycle for urea synthesis, ornithine transcarbamylase. What significance this may have will be discussed in Chapter 5. As in the case of arginase, the ornithine transaminase isoenzymes occurring in the various tissues appear to be so individually regulated that it will be most convenient to consider each separately.

It has been suggested that the hepatic isoenzyme is concerned primarily with the synthesis and catabolism of ornithine and arginine and with the regulation of the ornithine cycle, whereas the renal isoenzyme is more closely involved with synthesis of glutamate and proline. On the other hand, it is believed by some that the transaminase is important in ornithine biosynthesis in whatever tissue it occurs, and that it is rate-limiting in that process in each case.

In consonance with its possible anaplerotic role in the ornithine cycle, hepatic ornithine transaminase levels are increased on high-protein diets or by administration of amino acid mixtures, by glucagon, and in experimental diabetes (all of which conditions are characterized by increased rates of gluconeogenesis and protein catabolism), whereas decreases are seen with increased carbohydrate in the diet, administration of growth hormone, and in regenerating liver (conditions of decreased gluconeogenesis and increased protein anabolism). In contrast to these observations, other regulatory effects either militate against, or at least are completely independent of, the participation of the transaminase in the ornithine cycle. Thus, the induction by a high-protein diet appears to be restricted to relatively young animals, the increased levels in diabetes are not correlated with any direct effect of insulin, and fasting results in an anomalous fall in the total enzyme content of liver. Miscellaneous effects include the induction of the enzyme by specific amino acids (see Fig. 4-10) and estrogens and the discordant effects of arginine, which has been reported to act as an inducer in certain test systems and as a repressor in others. In common with the isoenzymes of all other tissues tested, hepatic ornithine transaminase activity is inhibited by branched-chain amino acids.

The effects of glucocorticoid hormones are altogether puzzling. On the one hand, glucocorticoid inhibits the induction of the enzyme by high-protein diets; on the other, the repressive effect of glucose upon the induction by high-protein diets or glucagon is counteracted by glucocorticoid. Attempts have been made to simplify the experimental situation by eliminating the influence of both pituitary and pancreatic hormones through combined hypophysectomy-pancreatectomy. In such rats, the transaminase is induced only slightly by glucagon alone and inconsistently by cAMP or its derivatives alone, whereas large inductive effects are produced by both factors when administered along with glucocorticoid hormones. Glucocorticoid alone is inconsistent in inducing ornithine transaminase in rats of the age usually used, but it is effective in pancreatectomized younger rats. It is probable that glucocorticoid itself has a true inductive effect in younger animals, a response lost with increasing age, the residual function of such hormones then becoming the permissive type.

In the development of the rat, hepatic ornithine transaminase increases in level transiently at birth, but in general parallels the development of the ornithine cycle enzymes during the weaning period. After birth of the rat but before the normal weaning-period rise, the hepatic transaminase may be prematurely evoked by administration of glucocorticoids, an effect which is repressible by estrogen. Estrogen also can block the normal developmental increase.

Although renal ornithine transaminase resembles its hepatic isoenzyme in decreasing in level during fasting, it is uninfluenced by the protein content of the diet, and increases in level in response to carbohydrate administration. Inductive effects also are shown by estrogen (much greater effect than in liver), branched-chain amino acids, and methionine. The suggested role of the kidney enzyme in the arginine (ornithine) → glutamate conversion is perhaps supported by the inductive effect of ornithine and the repressive effect of glutamate.

The renal enzyme develops at about the same time as the hepatic, but with a somewhat different pattern in time. Final levels in the female kidney are higher than those in the liver or kidney of the male or in the liver of the female. In striking contrast to what was said in regard to the hepatic enzyme, estrogen acts as a potent developmental inducer of the transaminase in kidney, and its effects are counteracted by glucocorticoid.

Little is known of the regulation of ornithine transaminase in other tissues. The enzyme is induced in liver cell cultures by branched-chain amino acids, ornithine, arginine, homocysteine, and methionine, and repressed in HeLa cells by proline. The enzyme of the small intestine is not affected by the factors which control the hepatic or renal enzymes, except that all have in common the inhibition by branched-chain amino acids, a phenomenon of unknown physiological significance.

What can be concluded concerning the role of ornithine transaminase, especially in liver and kidney? From the reported regulatory effects, it is evident that the liver enzyme has multiple functions, as has been suggested. Some of these may be related to the operation of the ornithine cycle, some to the catabolism of arginine. As will be noted again in Chapter 5, it is probable that the latter of these two functions may be the more important, particularly in circumstances calling for increased degradation of, and gluconeogenesis from, arginine. (Much of the suggested relationship of ornithine transaminase to the ornithine cycle does not stand up well under detailed scrutiny.) Other functions of the liver enzyme, as well as those of the kidney enzyme, can only be guessed at for the present, but may well have to do with the interconversion of arginine and ornithine on the one side, with glutamate and proline on the other. What is clear is that, in this area, as well as in certain others in amino acid metabolism, observations have accumulated at a faster rate than the theories which are required to explain their meaning for intermediary metabolism and for the survival value of the organism.

HISTIDINE.   As indicated in Figure 4-11, the two catabolic pathways of histidine in the mammalian organism are initiated by histidine-pyruvate transaminase and by histidine-ammonia lyase (commonly called histidase). Although the total histidine transaminase activity (which exists in the form of mitochondrial and cytosolic isoenzymes) of liver exceeds that of histidase, the latter nevertheless represents the preferred route under normal circumstances. The transaminase pathway becomes the major route by default in the inborn error of histidinemia, in which condition histidase is absent.

Transamination of histidine is followed either by reduction of imidazolepyruvate to imidazolelactate, or by oxidative decarboxylation of the keto acid to imidazoleacetate. Neither product is known to be metabolized further in the mammal.

Histidase, first enzyme on the major catabolic pathway, represents one of only a few lyases occurring in the mammalian organism. The formation of free ammonia by a nonoxidative, nonhydrolytic reaction also is something of a rarity, although this distinction must be shared with the serine-threonine dehydratase. The urocanate which is produced by the histidase reaction undergoes hydration and rearrangement under the influence of urocanase to form the rather unstable imidazolonepropionate. This product is converted by a hydrolase to formiminoglutamate, the formimino group (one type of one-carbon fragment) of which becomes attached to tetrahydrofolate under the influence of a transferase.

Despite the absence of metabolites of the glucogenic, ketogenic, or generally ergogenic type, it has been found that histidine-pyruvate transaminase is subject to regulation, chiefly (with some exceptions) of the type characteristic of gluconeogenic pathways. The significance of this regulation is not understood at this time.

The mitochondrial isoenzyme of hepatic histidine transaminase is induced, along with that in the cytosol, by glucagon or cAMP. However, the magnitude of the effect is much greater on the soluble enzyme, which is also induced by glucocorticoids, agents having little or no effect on the mitochondrial transaminase. The soluble transaminase is increased in level following injection of large amounts of thyroxine. Measured without regard for the separate isoenzymes, but probably reflecting the soluble member of the pair, fasting and alloxan diabetes slightly increase the transaminase level, which is decreased by a low-protein diet or by adrenalectomy. A high-protein diet usually has been

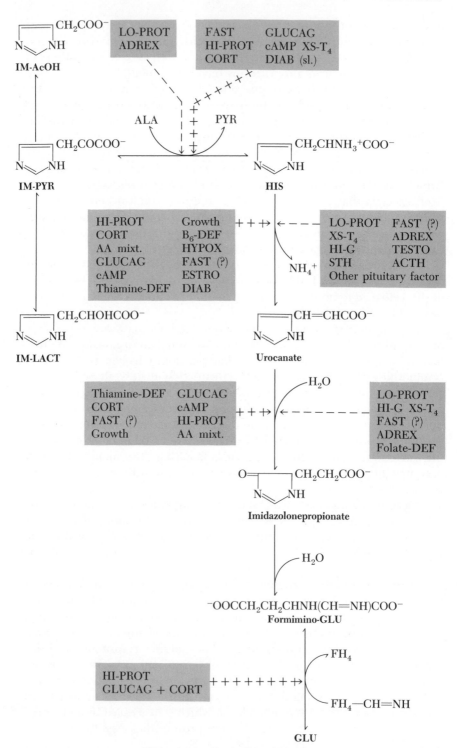

Figure 4–11. Catabolism of histidine.

reported to have an inductive effect, although one study found high levels of the enzyme produced at both high and low proportions of protein in the diet.

Developmental regulation of histidine-pyruvate transaminase may vary among species. The enzyme develops in the late fetal period in rats, whereas, based upon observations on imidazolepyruvate excretion in human histidinurics, the human neonate may have no significant transaminase activity for the first 6 or 7 weeks after birth.

Since both histidase and urocanase, the enzymes catalyzing the first and second steps, respectively, of the pathway to glutamate, lie on a gluconeogenic route, it is not unexpected to find that they are controlled by most of the usual dietary and endocrine factors. However, certain of their regulatory characteristics are atypical; for these we have no explanation at present.

Histidase is induced by a high-protein diet (or amino acid mixture), diabetes, glucocorticoids, glucagon, and cAMP, all of which are usual; but in addition, histidase is also induced by conditions of rapid growth, deficiency of pyridoxine or thiamine, hypophysectomy, and estrogen, none of which is typical of gluconeogenic pathways. Hypophysectomy is effective only in the male or ovariectomized female rat. The effect of estrogen, which will be discussed further in connection with developmental regulation, is indirect; it is believed to inhibit secretion of an hypophyseal suppressor of histidase. Contradictory results have been reported for the influence of fasting, probably due in part to the modest proportions of the effect, in part to its odd time-course, which appears as a slight rise followed by a more significant fall in level of the enzyme over the course of a week. Insulin and epinephrine are reported to have no effect upon the level of histidase in the liver.

Hepatic histidase levels are decreased by protein deficiency, thyroid hormones in excess, glucose, adrenalectomy, androgen, growth hormone, adrenocorticotropic hormone (acting extra-adrenally), and an as yet unidentified pituitary factor which is counteracted by estrogen. Androgen is not an independent repressor, but acts as an anti-estrogen. As in the case of the inducers, some of these repressors are typically gluconeogenic; others are peculiar to this area of histidine metabolism.

Histidase first appears in fetal rat liver shortly before birth, but at a very low level, its development occurring primarily in the weaning period. A second developmental phase takes place at puberty in both sexes, but the augmentation of enzyme content in the liver is much greater in the female, resulting in the adult female rat having twice the activity of the adult male rat. The difference is due to the secretion of estrogen in the female. It has been established, however, as mentioned earlier, that estrogen is not a direct inducer; rather it counteracts the repressing influence of a pituitary factor. The physiological significance of these endocrine controls on hepatic histidase is not known.

Urocanase, the second enzyme in the sequence under consideration, presents its own complement of regulatory factors in yet another example of regulatory redundancy. As in the case of the preceding enzyme, it will be seen that these factors comprise a mixed bag, partly gluconeogenic and partly idiosyncratic.

Among the inducers of urocanase may be listed glucocorticoids, glucagon, cAMP, high-protein diet or amino acid mixture, conditions of rapid growth, and thiamine deficiency. Repressing influences are exerted by adrenalectomy, glucose, low-protein diet, excessive amounts of thyroid hormones, and folic-acid deficiency. As was mentioned in connection with histidase, contradictory results have been reported for the effects of fasting. Developmentally, urocanase belongs to the late fetal period.

There has been little reported of a regulatory nature concerning the two reactions following urocanase. Preliminary observations indicate that the formimino-transferase is induced by a high-protein diet and by administration of a combination of glucagon and glucocorticoid.

Finally, it may be noted that, although the transaminase and the histidase pathways of histidine catabolism both appear to be susceptible to *qualitatively* similar gluconeogenic influences, significant *quantitative* differences have been observed. Thus, the soluble transaminase is very much more responsive to the inductive influences of glucagon and glucocorticoid than are histidase and urocanase, whereas exactly the opposite obtains in the case of a high-protein diet.

What can be concluded about the overall role of regulation of histidine metabolism (at least that phase of it treated in this chapter)? For one thing, it does not appear that histidine is a major source of raw material for gluconeogenesis; the developmental characteristics of the chief enzymes of histidine catabolism, their unimpressive behavior during fasting, and their anomalous response to conditions of growth all militate against such a role. Of course, the first three enzymes discussed in this section are not noted for their rapid response to most inductive or repressive influences, behavior made understandable by the finding that the half-lives of these enzymes, under various conditions of induction or repression, are in the range of 3 to 5 days. Perhaps those gluconeogenic factors which do influence the histidine-catabolizing enzymes are vestiges of an earlier era in evolution. For the other numerous odd regulators which influence this pathway, no physiological justification has been proffered in the literature.

PROLINE AND HYDROXYPROLINE.   The major pathway for anabolism and catabolism of proline is shown in Figure 4-12. As indicated earlier, although the catabolism of hydroxyproline eventuates in pyruvate rather than ketoglutarate (or glutamate), it is included in this section because its metabolic route closely parallels that of proline. In fact, except for the last two catabolic reactions illustrated in the hydroxyproline sequence, identical enzymes are involved.

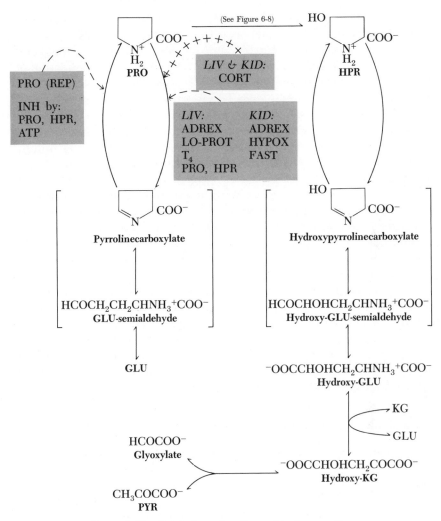

Figure 4–12. Catabolism of proline and hydroxyproline.

Proline is oxidized, in both liver and kidney, by a mitochondrial proline oxidase system (which is irreversible) to pyrrolinecarboxylate, which exists in rapid nonenzymatic equilibrium with the open-chain glutamate semialdehyde. The reverse reaction is catalyzed by another enzyme, a soluble NADH-utilizing reductase. Glutamate semialdehyde is reversibly oxidized to glutamate by a mitochondrial dehydrogenase.

Hydroxyproline undergoes parallel reactions. The hydroxyglutamate which is produced in this route is transaminated to hydroxyketoglutarate, which is cleaved by an aldolase to glyoxylate and pyruvate.

Proline is converted to hydroxyproline by proline hydroxylase, which, however, will not be discussed in this section, since the properties of this enzyme are more closely related to the synthesis of collagen than to the general anabolic or catabolic reactions of the prolines.

Despite the long-recognized glucogenicity of both proline and hydroxyproline, there has been relatively little study of the regulation of this pathway, as can be seen in Figure 4-12. The biosynthesis of proline from carbohydrate-related metabolites in various human cell cultures is repressed by the presence of proline. In cultures of L-cells (mouse fibroblasts) this repression has been localized at the pyrrolinecarboxylate reductase step. The activity of the reductase is inhibited by ATP and by the prolines, but in the latter cases only at unphysiologically high concentrations.

There is some disagreement in the literature concerning the similarity (or dissimilarity) in the regulatory characteristics of the proline oxidase of liver and kidney. In general, this enzyme appears to be induced by glucocorticoids, repressed by adrenalectomy, hypophysectomy, fasting, protein deficiency, hyperthyroidism, and intraperitoneal administration of the prolines. In the liver of the rat, seasonal variations in activity are considerable. Despite the apparent identity of the enzymes involved in the metabolism of the prolines, one report states that hydroxyproline oxidation in liver is unresponsive to regulation by glucocorticoids, thyroid hormones, or administration of prolines.

A certain resemblance to the metabolism of histidine is evident in the preceding, in that controlling factors of the gluconeogenic type are admixed with others having no relationship to such a pathway.

The Ketobutyrate Family of Amino Acids

METHIONINE.   Although methionine is involved in many different metabolic reactions (e.g., transmethylations), the pathway which accounts for most of this amino acid which is turned over per day is the reaction sequence in which the sulfur of methionine is incorporated into cysteine and the carbon chain into alpha-ketobutyrate. This pathway, which consists of two initial reactions catalyzed by cystathionine synthase and cystathionase, respectively, is illustrated in Figure 4-13. Contrary to earlier beliefs, the synthase is not identical with serine dehydratase. Cystathionase, however, is the same enzyme as cysteine desulfhydrase, which was discussed in the section on cysteine. Both enzymes are soluble and require pyridoxal phosphate as coenzyme.

Although the ketobutyrate produced from methionine (and from threonine) is a glucogenic compound, being readily decarboxylated to propionate, which in turn forms succinate in several steps, methionine has not been shown to be unequivocally glucogenic by the classic techniques. Thus, it does not form significant amounts of glycogen when administered to the fasted animal, but has been reported to produce extra urinary glucose in the experimentally diabetic. The overall rate of con-

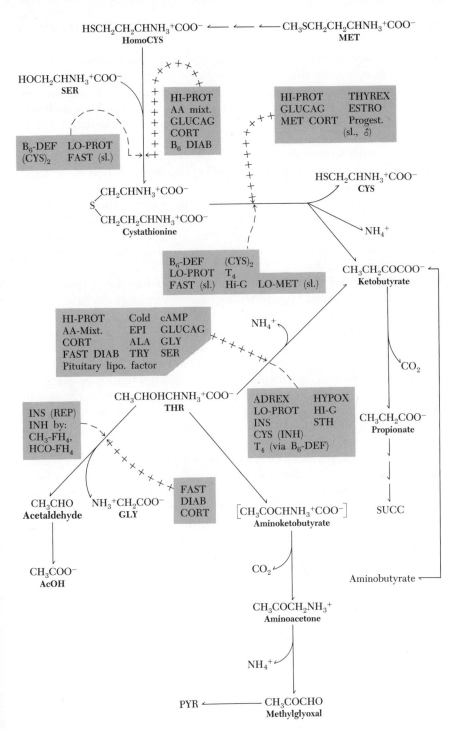

Figure 4–13. Major hepatic catabolic pathways of methionine and threonine.

version of methionine to ketobutyrate may be too slow to form glucose rapidly enough to be detectable under all test conditions.

Homocysteine, the demethylated derivative of methionine, rather than methionine itself, is the initial compound on the catabolic pathway. It can be derived from methionine by activation of the latter (as in preparation for transmethylations) through interaction with ATP, forming S-adenosylmethionine. Following transmethylation, the residual S-adenosylhomocysteine loses its adenosyl group by hydrolysis to yield the desired product.

As indicated in Figure 4-13, both cystathionine synthase and cystathionase of liver are induced by high-protein diets, glucagon, and glucocorticoids, and repressed by pyridoxine deficiency, low-protein diets, inclusion of cystine in the diet, and (contrary to most gluconeogenic pathways) by fasting. The synthase itself is additionally induced by pyridoxine and the diabetic condition. Cystathionase is induced by methionine, estrogens, progesterone, and thyroidectomy and is repressed by thyroid hormones and glucose.

Not indicated in the figure are reports on the synthase, disagreeing on the effects of diabetes on the liver enzyme, and showing for the kidney enzyme repression by diabetes, thyroid hormones, and testosterone. Cystathionase in liver, according to some, is not influenced by glucocorticoids, adrenalectomy, or fasting and is actually slightly decreased in level on a high-protein diet. Renal cystathionase is said to be increased in level by thyroid hormones and low-protein diets, and decreased in diabetes.

Developmentally, both enzymes have significant (but less than adult) activity in the liver of the suckling rat and in the full-term newborn human. The human fetus and premature infant have the synthase, but lack the cystathionase. This last observation suggests that cysteine may be an essential amino acid in the human under conditions of premature birth. An interesting example of species differences is provided by the finding that cystathionase is present in the liver of the rat fetus on the twelfth day of gestation.

If one ignores the occasional contradictory reports in the literature, and holds in abeyance any conclusions concerning the regulation of methionine catabolism in kidney until more is known of its role, then most of the regulatory factors affecting the two hepatic enzymes are those characteristic of gluconeogenic (and related) pathways. The chief exception is fasting, which has a negative (albeit small) effect on the levels of both enzymes.

The repressive influence of cystine upon the thionase and, even more strongly, on the synthase seems to represent a good mammalian example of metabolite repression of an early enzyme in a sequence. In addition, there is provided a molecular basis for the *in vivo* observation that inclusion of cystine in the diet spares a portion of the daily requirement for methionine, since, in the presence of the nonessential amino acid, a catabolic pathway for destruction of an essential amino acid is switched off.

THREONINE.   In the scheme for threonine catabolism, included also in Figure 4-13, it will be noted that one of the three pathways depicted leads to the formation of ketobutyrate, the chief justification for considering the catabolism of threonine along with that of methionine. Mechanistically speaking, threonine could as easily have been considered along with serine, since two of the pathways of the former utilize enzymes which are apparently identical with two enzymes which attack the latter.

Since threonine aldolase is identical with serine aldolase (also called serine transhydroxymethylase), and since threonine dehydratase is identical, in most species, with serine dehydratase, regulatory factors for both of these enzymes have been transferred bodily from Figures 4-8 and 4-9 to Figure 4-13. In both earlier and later figures, data obtained with either serine or threonine have been combined.

Threonine sometimes has been classified as a glucogenic amino acid, since it has been reported to form liver glycogen in the fasted rat. In agreement with this, the dehydratase pathway, yielding ketobutyrate, probably constitutes the chief avenue of threonine catabolism. It will be noted that the regulation of this pathway is characteristic of gluconeogenic routes.

The aminoacetone pathway of threonine catabolism, which begins with the action of the mitochondrial threonine dehydrogenase, also is glucogenic, terminating in pyruvate (see analogous pathway involving aminoacetone from glycine). Unfortunately, nothing is known of its regulation. It is believed, however, to account for only a minor fraction of the daily turnover of threonine.

From the standpoint of one of the leading arguments of this monograph, the aldolase pathway is particularly interesting. This route (which accounts for a substantial fraction of total threonine degradation) gives rise to glycine, a dubiously glucogenic compound, and acetaldehyde, an acetogenic and ketogenic metabolite. The regulatory factors, fasting, diabetes, and glucocorticoids on the positive side, and insulin on the negative side, are evidently at least as important for acetoneogenesis as for pyruvoneogenesis. Further examples of this phenomenon will come to light later in this chapter, when more frankly ketogenic amino acids are discussed. Inhibition of the aldolase by methyl- and formyl-tetrahydrofolate may be due, as in the analogous reaction with serine, to negative feedback by metabolite, since glycine, one of the products of the reaction with threonine, is a source of one-carbon fragments.

Branched-chain Amino Acids

Abbreviated versions of the catabolic pathways of leucine, isoleucine, and valine are given in Figure 4-14.

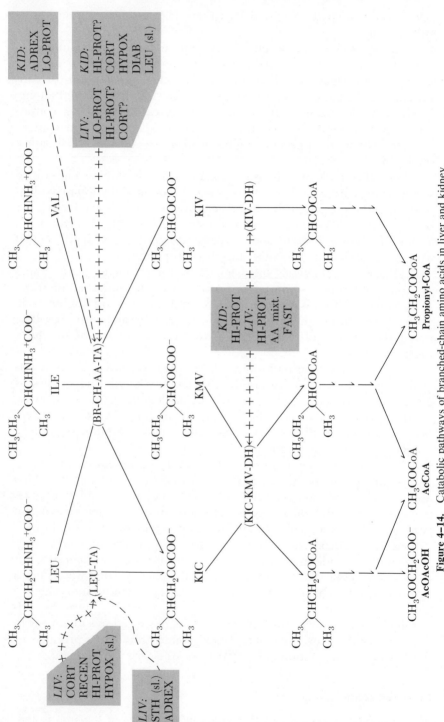

Figure 4-14. Catabolic pathways of branched-chain amino acids in liver and kidney.

Catabolism of the branched-chain amino acids begins with trans-amination (involving ketoglutarate). The resulting keto acids are oxidatively decarboxylated to the coenzyme-A thioesters of the acids of one less carbon atom. By additional reactions, also remarkably similar in the three pathways, leucine yields two ketogenic fragments (acetoacetate and acetyl-CoA), valine one glucogenic fragment (propionyl-CoA), and isoleucine a pair consisting of one fragment of each type.

The parallelism in reaction types undergone by the intermediates of the three amino acids led, naturally, to suggestions that the same enzyme catalyzed this or that reaction of all three pathways. The idea was reinforced by the occurrence of an inborn error of metabolism, maple syrup urine disease or branched-chain ketoaciduria, in which a blockade appeared to exist simultaneously in all three pathways. Recent investigations seem to be indicating that, for the transamination and oxidative decarboxylation steps, there are indeed enzymes of broader specificity, but occurring along with others of narrow specificity. Intra- and extramitochondrial isoenzymes frequently exist, each with its characteristic response to regulatory influences, which in turn may differ from one tissue to another.

As noted earlier in this monograph (Chapter 2), there is much evidence that, in contrast to other amino acids, the catabolism of the branched-chain group occurs chiefly outside the liver. In agreement with this, surveys of transaminase activity for the branched-chain amino acids in the rat have yielded the highest values in heart and kidney, intermediate in skeletal muscle, and lowest in liver. The physiological significance of this difference in chief catabolic sites for different groups of amino acids is not apparent at this time. Nevertheless, since the liver is equipped with a full complement of catabolic enzymes for the branched-chain amino acids, and since the regulation of these pathways in liver seems to have certain characteristics of its own, and especially since there are papers published on it, liver will be considered along with kidney and other tissues.

A general branched-chain amino acid transaminase, working equally well with leucine, isoleucine, and valine, is widely distributed in animal tissues. Isoenzymic forms occur in mitochondria and in the cytosol, with the latter accounting for most of the activity of the cell. In addition, a specific leucine transaminase is found in rat liver, possibly a species idiosyncrasy, since it does not occur in hog tissues. Although most of the activity of this transaminase is confined to the mitochondria, an isoenzyme is found also in the cytosol. Brain cytosol appears to contain a third type of branched-chain amino acid transaminase, its properties differing somewhat from those of the nearly ubiquitous first enzyme mentioned above.

Although it is generally accepted that the level of the cytosolic, specific leucine transaminase of rat liver varies with the protein level of the diet, one laboratory has reported that the total transamination of leucine (presumably consisting of that due to the leucine transaminase plus that due to the enzyme of broader specificity) is affected by the protein content of the diet only in the case of the mitochondrial activity, not the soluble. The soluble leucine transaminase is induced also by glucocorticoids, in regenerating liver, and slightly after hypophysectomy. It is repressed by adrenalectomy and slightly by administration of growth hormone. Treatment with insulin, glucagon, or fasting is reported to have no effect on this transaminase. Rat liver leucine transaminase appears to have a more rapid rate of turnover than the general branched-chain amino acid transaminase of rat kidney. The former generally exhibits significant responses to inducers within a matter of hours to 1 day, whereas the latter may require several days to 2 weeks.

Controversy also characterizes the results concerning regulation of the general branched-chain amino acid transaminase. According to one laboratory, this enzyme in liver does not respond to regulators. In kidney it is induced by glucocorticoids and the diabetic state, but not by high-protein diets. The kidney enzyme is decreased by adrenalectomy. Another group reports that the same enzyme is induced by high-protein diets in liver, kidney, and muscle, whereas protein deficiency causes an increase in liver and muscle levels, and a decrease in kidney. Glucocorticoids, upon repeated administration for several days, induce the enzyme in liver and muscle, but not in kidney. Hypophysectomy is said to increase the level of the renal enzyme. Feeding of leucine does the same to a slight extent.

In the liver cytosol of the rat fetus (probably late in gestation), only the general branched-chain amino acid transaminase is found. This enzyme falls in level at around birth, then decreases even further toward adulthood. In contrast, the leucine transaminase found in this species does not appear until after birth, and should be classified in the neonatal developmental group. The general relationship of the leucine enzyme to the growth process is obscure; it is induced in regenerating rat liver beginning 6 hours after operation, remains at a high level for another 6 hours, then decreases to normal, all of these events taking place well before the increase in cell division. Adrenalectomy reduces but does not eliminate the regenerative induction.

Considerably less controversy surrounds the enzymes catalyzing the oxidative decarboxylation of the keto acid products of the transaminases. The reaction is catalyzed by dehydrogenases which are chiefly mitochondrial. Although those of rat tissues are thus far not separable, in other species (e.g., bovine liver) a dehydrogenase specific for ketoisovalerate (from valine) has been separated from another with double specificity toward ketoisocaproate (from leucine) and ketomethylvalerate (from isoleucine).

Despite the existence of two distinct enzymes catalyzing the reaction, it has been shown that, under the influence of various regulatory factors, the mitochondrial dehydrogenase activity toward all three keto acids rises and falls in concert. In addition, in branched-chain ketoaciduria, cultured cells from the affected patients are defective in oxidation of all three keto acids. Since the enzymes in question are not simple dehydrogenases, but rather dehydrogenase systems analogous to those catalyzing the oxidative decarboxylations of pyruvate and ketoglutarate in mitochondria, it is quite possible that at least one of the several protein components of the complex is common to the two enzymes. This would explain a simultaneous genetic defect in the two systems, and, if the shared component were the regulated site, the instances of concerted induction as well.

High-protein diets induce higher levels of the dehydrogenases in liver and (slightly) in kidney. The liver enzymes are increased also by fasting and by administration of amino acids. Although tested originally with branched-chain amino acids, the latter effect is not specific for only this one type of amino acid. It is of interest that the high-protein induction reaches a plateau at about 30 per cent casein (in the rat), which has led to the hypothesis that this particular regulatory mechanism may not have as its chief function the role of allowing the animal to handle very large loads of protein, but rather of decreasing the rate of catabolism of a group of essential amino acids when the protein intake is low.

The branched-chain keto acid dehydrogenases of bovine liver are activated *in vitro* by inorganic phosphate and Ca^{++} and are inhibited by ATP. Whether these effects are physiologically significant, and whether they represent regulatory mechanisms directed specifically at the dehydrogenases or are concerned more closely with the properties of the mitochondrial membranes are questions which cannot be answered as yet.

The hepatic dehydrogenases of the rat exhibit a circadian rhythm, which is not triggered by the ingestion of food. Little developmental information on the dehydrogenases has been reported. In the guinea pig, the overall decarboxylation of the carboxyl group of leucine (isotopically labeled), which includes the transamination step, occurs in midgestation as well as in the near-term fetus.

At this time it appears impossible to reconcile the flatly contradictory findings reported for the branched-chain amino acid transaminases. What is of interest is that most of the reported regulatory influences, whether confirmed by another laboratory or not, do not depart from the usual gluconeogenic controls. Since these are herein applied to pathways giving rise to ketogenic and glucogenic fragments alike, it is evident that we have strong support for one of the chief arguments of this monograph, namely that the metabolic signal characterized by a certain set of regulators represents, not simply a specific call for glucose-formation as such, but also a demand for extra energy production (ergoneogenesis), with the machinery of the cells oxidizing whatever can be mobilized.

Lysine

What little is known of the regulation of lysine catabolism is illustrated in Figure 4-15. It will be noted that two pathways are depicted, at least for the initial few reactions; both merge in aminoadipate-semialdehyde. Until just a few years ago, the pathway through pipecolate was regarded as the chief, if not the only, route of degradation of lysine. Current opinion, backed by substantial evidence, favors the route through saccharopine, that involving pipecolate being relegated to, at best, minor status. As a matter of curiosity, it may be seen that the two-step synthesis and cleavage of saccharopine accomplish the same end as a simple transamination. Why evolution has favored the more complex mechanism is unclear.

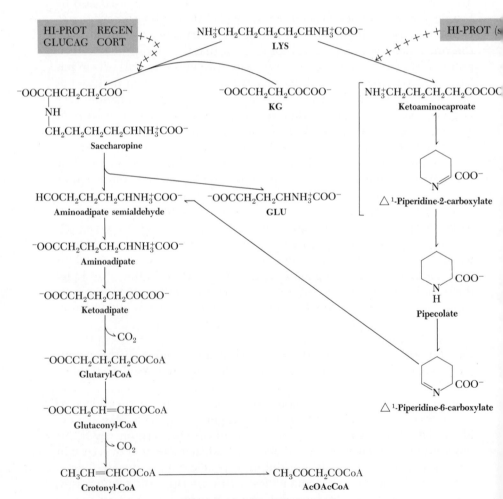

Figure 4–15.   Catabolism of lysine.

Although Ringer in 1912 reported that glutarate (then, as now, regarded as a metabolite of lysine) slightly increased the hydroxybutyrate output in the urine of a phlorizin-diabetic dog, most classic balance studies have failed to furnish evidence that lysine is either ketogenic or glucogenic. The more modern studies which conclude that a molecule of acetoacetate is formed from each molecule of lysine degraded can be reconciled with the older work on the assumption that the *rate* of production of ketone bodies is insufficient to yield positive results by other than isotopic labeling methods.

Unpublished work quoted in a recent review indicates the existence in adult (not fetal) liver of an NAD-linked lysine dehydrogenase attacking the alpha-amino group. This enzyme, which presumably is connected with the pipecolate route, is increased in level slightly on a high-protein diet.

The conversion of lysine to saccharopine, probably reflecting the activity of the lysine-ketoglutarate reductase, increases in the liver regenerating after partial hepatectomy, the general pattern in time being similar to that of the leucine transaminase discussed in the previous section. The overall oxidation of the carboxyl carbon of lysine to CO_2, again believed to be limited by the activity of the saccharopine-forming enzyme, is increased by a high-protein diet and administration of glucagon or glucocorticoids, the actions of the two types of hormones being synergistic when given simultaneously.

It is evident that we have here again an example of classically gluconeogenic controls over an essentially ketogenic route.

Tryptophan

The major catabolic pathways of tryptophan are shown in Figure 4-16. Several minor branches of these pathways are omitted for simplification. The chief catabolic route is initiated by the conversion of tryptophan to formylkynurenine, catalyzed by tryptophan oxygenase (more commonly called tryptophan pyrrolase), located in the cytosol. The pyrrolase, a heme-enzyme, is distinguished from others of its kind by the ease of dissociation of its prosthetic group. The pyrrolase is notable also for the amount of study expended on its regulatory properties since its inducibility was discovered by Knox in 1951.

Following loss of the formyl group (cytosolic formamidase), kynurenine is oxidized by a mitochondrial hydroxylase. Kynureninase (cytosolic), which can also attack unhydroxylated kynurenine to initiate one of the omitted side paths, removes an alanine moiety to yield hydroxyanthranilate. Despite formation of an ordinarily glucogenic fragment, tryptophan is not glucogenic by the classic criteria, probably due to the rather small amount catabolized per day. In addition, tryptophan, through one of its metabolites, quinolinate, acts as an inhibitor of

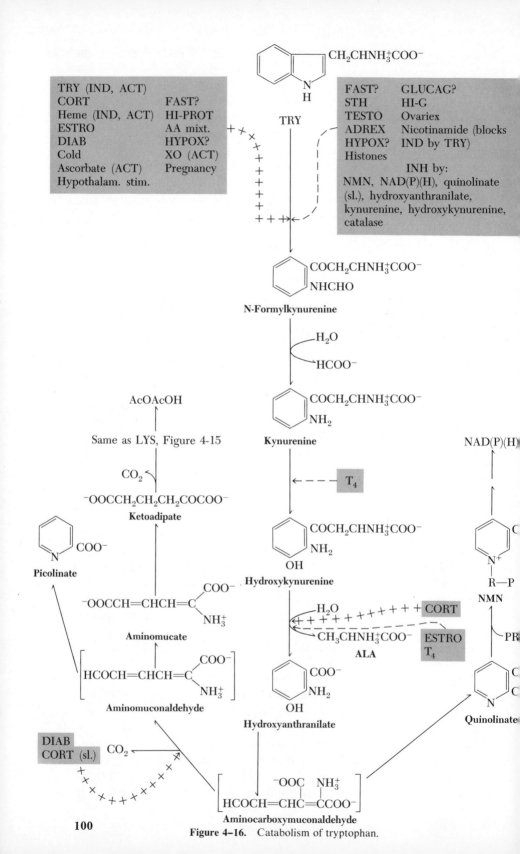

Figure 4-16. Catabolism of tryptophan.

gluconeogenesis. The affected enzyme is phosphoenolpyruvate carboxy-kinase.

Hydroxylation of hydroxyanthranilate, accompanied by cleavage of the aromatic ring, produces a labile intermediate (aminocarboxymucon-aldehyde) which stands at a crossroads in tryptophan metabolism. The quantitatively most important route involves decarboxylation (picolinate carboxylase) to yield another labile intermediate, aminomuconaldehyde. A minor branch of this pathway follows cyclization of this intermediate to picolinate, a metabolic cul-de-sac. The main route leads through adipate and glutarate derivatives, terminating, as does the similar pathway of lysine catabolism, in acetoacetate. It may be noted that tryptophan is not demonstrably ketogenic, probably for the same reason that it is not glucogenic.

If aminocarboxymuconaldehyde, instead of immediate decarboxylation, first undergoes cyclization, forming quinolinate, the latter may be coupled with phosphoribosyl pyrophosphate to initiate a pathway which leads to the formation of NAD and related nucleotide coenzymes, all derivatives of the vitamin, nicotinamide. This formation of a vitamin from an amino acid is unique in the animal organism, and accounts for the observation that provision of adequate amounts of tryptophan in the diet reduces the requirement for the vitamin.

Tryptophan pyrrolase is induced by most of the usual glucogenic or, more properly, ergogenic agents, as can be seen in Figure 4-16. It should be noted, however, that considerable species differences exist, even among the mammals. There is indirect evidence that the enzyme in human liver resembles that in rat liver, with which most investigators have worked. Rabbit and mouse liver pyrrolases also probably belong to this group. In contrast, in cats, substrate induction is less evident than in rats, and induction by glucocorticoids is absent. Guinea pig liver pyrrolase is induced by substrate, but not by glucocorticoids. Neither type of induction appears to function in cattle or sheep.

Induction of tryptophan pyrrolase by tryptophan and by glucocorticoid hormones has been investigated in such detail that these phenomena will be discussed separately, after consideration of the actions of other agents, of both positive and negative influence.

The pyrrolase is reported to be induced by estrogens, the diabetic state, exposure to cold, pregnancy, a high-protein diet, administration of protein hydrolysate after protein depletion (with some disagreement), hypophysectomy (with controversy), and electrical stimulation of the hypothalamus. Although most investigators report induction by fasting, lowering of enzyme level has been found in one laboratory. It may be noted that, in contrast to most of the regulated amino acid catabolizing enzymes discussed in this monograph, the pyrrolase is not induced by glucagon; indeed, one laboratory reports lower levels of the enzyme after administration of the hormone. Increasing the level of heme in the liver by induction of aminolevulinate synthase (see Chapter 6) results also in increasing the level of the pyrrolase, a cofactor type of induction (the *activating* effect of heme will be discussed shortly). Unphysiologically high doses of insulin, sufficient to cause convulsions in rats, increase the level of the pyrrolase, even after administration of glucose to prevent hypoglycemia.

Activation of the pyrrolase, which will be discussed in greater detail subsequently, can be effected by tryptophan, heme, and reducing agents such as ascorbate or peroxide (provided in the cell by xanthine oxidase), this last-named agent being counteracted, probably physiologically, by catalase. Additional natural activators of unknown identity exist in the microsomal and mitochondrial fractions of rat liver.

Decreases in the level of tryptophan pyrrolase in liver are seen after adrenalectomy, hypophysectomy (with some disagreement in the literature), treatment with growth hormone, injection of histones, treatment of female rats by ovariectomy or with androgen, or, as mentioned previously, according to one laboratory, by fasting or glucagon. The induction of the pyrrolase which follows induction of aminolevulinate synthase is blocked by prior administration of glucose, which also appears to act as a general repressor of the enzyme. Administration of nicotinamide, which raises the hepatic level of NAD, represses the tryptophan-mediated (but not the glucocorticoid-mediated) induction of the pyrrolase. In an example of negative feedback inhibition by metabolite, the *activity* of tryptophan pyrrolase is inhibited by NADPH (and by other tryptophan and nicotinamide derivatives) in the physiological range of concentration.

Returning now to the inductions of tryptophan pyrrolase by substrate and glucocorticoid hormones, Figure 4-17 illustrates the current status, factual and hypothetical, concerning these two forms of regulation. Although occasional disagreement has been voiced, it is generally agreed that induction by glucocorticoid and induction by tryptophan both are blocked by puromycin, whereas actinomycin D blocks only the former. Hence, in accord with what was discussed earlier in this monograph concerning sites of action of inhibitors of protein synthesis, the hormonal induction is presumed to function at the level of transcription (DNA to RNA) or, in certain more recent versions, at a later but still pretranslational level, whereas substrate induction is judged to take place at the level of translation. Immunochemical and isotope-labeling techniques have shown that glucocorticoid hormones increase the rate of synthesis of enzyme protein without affecting the rate of degradation. Induction of pyrrolase by substrate, on the other hand, operates exclusively by decreasing the rate of degradation.

Due to its dissociability, as much as two-thirds of the tryptophan pyrrolase in the average rat liver cell may be unsaturated with its heme cofactor. Induction by tryptophan takes place in stages and appears to

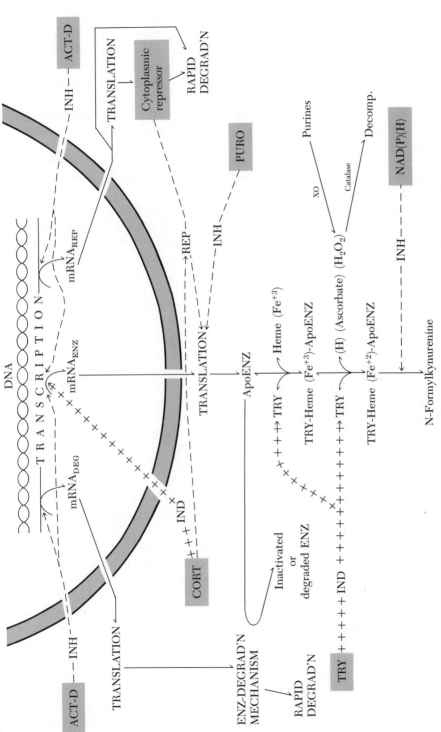

Figure 4–17. Regulation of tryptophan pyrrolase by substrate and glucocorticoids.

be a combination of activation and true increase in the total concentration of holoenzyme. In the first phase, apopyrrolase combines with ferric heme (hematin), a process which is favored by the presence of tryptophan, which probably exerts an allosteric influence upon the protein and may well combine with it also at this stage. This first phase also may be facilitated by increasing the concentration of heme in the cytoplasm (cofactor induction), an effect which can be achieved indirectly by inducing synthesis of the rate-limiting enzyme of porphyrin synthesis, aminolevulinate synthase.

In a second step, the catalytically inactive ferric form of the substrate-holoenzyme complex is reduced to the active ferrous form. (It should be noted that some investigators regard the oxidized form of the holoenzyme as an artifact of experimental manipulation, not as a stage in the physiological sequence of activation.) Reduction may be accomplished by ascorbate or by hydrogen peroxide, the latter being provided by the action of xanthine oxidase upon purines in the cell. The reduction also is facilitated by the presence of tryptophan. Several investigators have reported the presence in the cell of proteins which inhibit activation or induction of the pyrrolase. In a number of cases, this material has been identified as catalase, which may have a physiological function in preserving the metabolic balance, by destroying the hydrogen peroxide required in this and perhaps other systems.

The ferric and ferrous forms of the holopyrrolase are in equilibrium with the unconjugated apopyrrolase. In artificial degradative systems, the apopyrrolase has proved to be more labile than the holoenzyme, supporting the contention that enzymes in general are less labile when combined with cofactors, substrates, or both. Indeed, this mechanism often is presumed to be the way in which substrates and cofactors exert their inductive effects.

Induction of the pyrrolase by tryptophan, then, is believed to involve the following sequence. An influx of tryptophan into the liver cell first increases the rate of conjugation of apoenzyme with heme and the subsequent reduction. The ratio of activated to inactive pyrrolase is thus increased. As a consequence of the lower concentration of apoenzyme, the rate of degradation of pyrrolase is decreased. Hence, even with no increase in the absolute rate of synthesis of apoenzyme, an increased concentration of this protein will be detected, indicating induction at the translational level. Actual acceleration of translational events on the ribosome, although possibly resulting from the presence of substrate or cofactor (as noted in Chapter 1), apparently does not occur in the pyrrolase system.

There is considerably less agreement concerning the mechanism of induction of tryptophan pyrrolase by glucocorticoid hormones. According to one viewpoint, the hormones, either directly or through some intermediary agent from the cytosol (such as the steroid-receptor complex discussed in Chapter 1), exert an effect at the site of transcription, whereby, if a negative type of control system is involved, a repressor is derepressed, thus allowing an increased rate of coding of messenger RNA for pyrrolase from the genomic DNA. It is this transcription which is interfered with by actinomycin.

Unfortunately, this relatively simple scheme cannot explain all of the more recent experimental findings. One particularly vexing phenomenon is the so-called paradoxical action of actinomycin, in which, depending upon the specific test system, long-term dosage with the inhibitor, use of unusually high concentrations, or careful timing with relation to previously administered glucocorticoid results in a degree of induction well beyond that anticipated from the inductive agent itself, *superinduction.* Although attempts have been made to explain superinduction by actinomycin-inhibition of transcription of a messenger RNA for some protein component of the degradative system which inactivates the enzyme, instances are known in which no decrease in degradation can be detected.

One model which has been constructed to fit the above observations postulates the existence of a cytoplasmic repressor, protein in nature, the mRNA of which is prevented from being transcribed by actinomycin under the special circumstances mentioned previously. This repressor, which is postulated to be constantly and rapidly degraded, ordinarily prevents (or at least decreases the rate of) translation of pyrrolase mRNA on the ribosome, possibly by rendering this latter mRNA more susceptible to degradation. In any case, the glucocorticoid inducer, in addition to its nuclear activities, is believed to antagonize the antitranslational action of the cytoplasmic repressor. Later versions of this model confine the actions of the glucocorticoid hormone entirely to the cytoplasm.

It may be appropriate to terminate this discussion of induction of tryptophan pyrrolase with the thought, which has appeared intermittently throughout this monograph in various guises, that, although a mechanism may be shown to exist, it is another matter to show that it is used. To be more specific in this context, experiments with intact rats and with perfused rat livers have shown that, after induction of tryptophan pyrrolase, the rate of overall degradation of isotopically labeled tryptophan is not increased, or at least not in proportion to the extent of the induction. These observations suggest that the magnitude of tryptophan turnover may, under ordinary circumstances at least, be controlled by the load of amino acid presented to the cell. Perhaps variations in the concentration of enzyme represent a safety measure, a second line of defense.

There are few reports at hand on the regulation of steps subsequent to the pyrrolase along the major catabolic pathways for tryptophan. Excessive thyroxine reduces the level of kynurenine hydroxylase in rat liver mitochondria, along with that of several other enzymes (such as mono-amine oxidase) which accompany it in the outer membrane of the organelle. Kynureninase (which functions as a hydroxykynureninase in the major pathway) is induced by glucocorticoids, repressed by estrogen and thyroid hormones. Picolinate carboxylase is induced by glucocorticoids and diabetes.

Distinct species differences are seen in the developmental regulation of tryptophan pyrrolase. The enzyme is absent or present in only low concentration in fetal liver of all species tested. Although apparently present in most human newborns, the pyrrolase is absent in the premature infant. In the guinea pig and rabbit, the enzyme develops maximally in the neonatal period, reaching adult values during the first postnatal day. In contrast, rat liver pyrrolase has been variously reported as developing anywhere from the twelfth to the twenty-fourth day after birth, suggesting that its appearance may coincide with weaning.

Premature development of tryptophan pyrrolase by administration of tryptophan or glucocorticoids to the fetus has not succeeded. However, in rabbits, premature or postmature delivery immediately triggers postnatal development of the enzyme. In the 4-day-old rat, although neither tryptophan nor glucocorticoid alone will induce the pyrrolase, induction to the adult level in a period of only 5 hours can be evoked if injection of glucocorticoid is followed 1 day later by injection of tryptophan.

Development of the pyrrolase is blocked by puromycin, indicating involvement of the translation step of protein synthesis. Some investigators are of the opinion that development is largely substrate-controlled, since it is unaffected by adrenalectomy (at the age of 14 days) or actinomycin; others report inhibition of development of the enzyme by fluorouracil, which blocks transcription. From the induction of the pyrrolase prematurely by the sequential treatments with glucocorticoid and tryptophan referred to in the previous paragraph, and from the reported sensitivity of the hormonal phase only of this sequence to actinomycin, it seems likely that development of the pyrrolase is under controls of both the substrate and endocrine type, operating at both the transcriptional and translational levels.

In its postnatal spurt, tryptophan pyrrolase, in common with certain other enzymes, sometimes reaches levels well above those characteristic of the adult of the species. The significance of this "overshoot" phenomenon is not clear.

The turnover rate of the pyrrolase changes irregularly with increasing age. In the adult rat, the enzyme has a half-life of 2 to 3 hours.

Both the basal and the corticoid-induced levels of tryptophan pyrrolase are below normal in regenerating liver, which may be another facet of the general repressive effect of growth hormone upon the level of this enzyme.

Development of the formamidase (formylase) has been variously reported as late fetal or neonatal in the rat, late fetal in the guinea pig, and neonatal in the mouse. It cannot be induced prematurely by glucocorticoid.

Tryptophan pyrrolase is subject to a circadian rhythm, which, depending upon the reporting laboratory, is less intense but altered in timing after adrenalectomy, or abolished after adrenalectomy, or for which glucocorticoids are permissive but not essential. The rhythm appears to be independent of liver tryptophan or plasma glucocorticoid concentration. In contrast to tyrosine transaminase (which will be discussed later), the pyrrolase rhythm is affected only minimally by the timing of meals.

In summing up the regulatory characteristics of the major catabolic pathways of tryptophan, it is interesting to note two peculiarities. One is that, in contrast to most other amino acids, the focus of regulation in this case is on an enzyme which cleaves a heterocyclic ring, not on a deaminase. Another distinction is the complete insensitivity of the pyrrolase to the inductive influence of glucagon, which is effective in the case of the rate-limiting catabolic enzymes for so many other amino acids. Despite these exceptions, and the disagreements concerning the effects of fasting, tryptophan pyrrolase shares with most of the regulatory enzymes already discussed the capability of being induced by glucocorticoids, diabetes, and a high-protein diet and of being repressed by growth hormone.

Phenylalanine

As shown in Figure 4-18, the metabolism of phenylalanine, other than through conversion to tyrosine, is represented by a relatively small number of reactions. Transamination with either pyruvate or ketoglutarate yields phenylpyruvate, which may be reduced by an aromatic ketoacid reductase to phenyllactate, a metabolic end product which has no fate other than reoxidation. Alternately, phenylpyruvate may be oxidatively decarboxylated to phenylacetyl-CoA, some of which may be hydrolyzed to free phenylacetate, but most of which, in man, reacts with glutamine to form phenylacetylglutamine which is excreted in the urine. The foregoing pathways account for only a minor fraction of the daily turnover of phenylalanine under normal circumstances; they constitute a major fraction in the inborn error of metabolism, phenylketonuria.

The normally chief pathway of disposal of phenylalanine begins with its conversion to tyrosine. The direct catalyst of the reaction, an hydroxylase, utilizes atmospheric oxygen and, as cofactor, tetrahydrobiopterin, to replace the p-hydrogen atom on the benzene ring with an hydroxyl group. The oxidized pteridine is reduced by an auxiliary enzyme and NADPH. Mechanistically, the hydroxylation involves, not

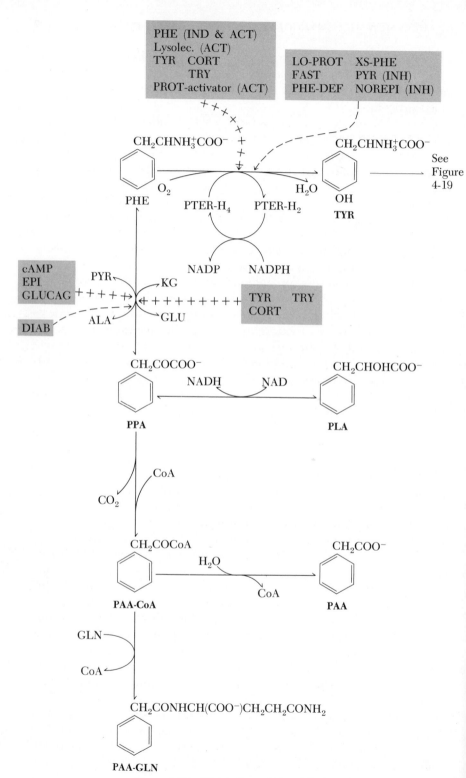

Figure 4–18. Metabolism of phenylalanine.

simple replacement of the *p*-hydrogen atom, but rather its transfer to an adjacent *m*-position, the so-called NIH shift, in the course of which a certain small amount of *m*-hydroxylation normally occurs also.

Although the phenylpyruvate pathway forms products which are not glucogenic, ketogenic, or, for that matter, ergogenic, it nevertheless appears to be subject to a certain amount of regulation. The hepatic level of the phenylalanine-ketoglutarate transaminase is increased by injection of tyrosine, tryptophan, or glucocorticoid, whereas that of the phenylalanine-pyruvate transaminase is increased by glucagon, epinephrine, and cAMP. The physiological significance of these controls is difficult to assess, especially in the case of the ketoglutarate enzyme. The properties of the phenylalanine-ketoglutarate transaminase may well be more accidental than biological, since it has been established that the *inducible* (but not the total) hepatic phenylalanine-ketoglutarate (as well as tryptophan-ketoglutarate) transaminase activity is due to the lack of specificity of the tyrosine-ketoglutarate transaminase to be discussed shortly.

Both phenylalanine transaminases are detectable in the late rat fetus but undergo their greatest developmental upsurge in the first day after birth.

Regulation of tyrosine formation from phenylalanine is directed at the hydroxylase proper, not at the auxiliary pteridine reductase, which in any case has a wider distribution than the hydroxylase and evidently subserves additional metabolic functions. The hydroxylase is induced by feeding of extra phenylalanine, tyrosine, or tryptophan and by administration of glucocorticoids. The *activity* of the hydroxylase is enhanced by phenylalanine, lysolecithin and certain other phospholipids, and by a protein activator found in liver, which probably shifts an association-dissociation equilibrium of the enzyme toward the monomeric form.

Hepatic levels of the hydroxylase are reduced by excess dietary phenylalanine, protein-depletion, phenylalanine-deficient diet (probably equivalent to protein depletion), and overnight fasting. A high-protein diet is reported to result in a slight and probably not significant decrease. The enzyme is inhibited by 10^{-4}M pyruvate, a factor which may be physiologically significant, and by a number of catecholamines.

Phenylalanine hydroxylase activity is low, but detectable, in the livers of most animal fetuses. Human fetuses contain the hydroxylase at 11 weeks of gestation. According to some, the low activity in the early phase of development is due largely to lack of the pteridine cofactor. The major increase in activity is neonatal; in the rat, a second increase occurs at weaning.

Rat liver hydroxylase exhibits a circadian rhythm which persists, albeit at a lower level of activity, during fasting. The rhythm is not correlated with the intake of phenylalanine.

Since conversion of phenylalanine to tyrosine opens to the former amino acid a pathway leading to the formation of both glucogenic (fumarate) and ketogenic (acetoacetate) fragments, the occurrence of at least some of the factors regulating the hydroxylase is not unexpected, examples being the effects of glucocorticoids and protein depletion. On the other hand, the biological *raisons d'être* for induction by the product tyrosine, for repression by the substrate phenylalanine, for the effect of fasting, or for the lack of effect of a high-protein diet all remain unknown.

Tyrosine

The major pathway of tyrosine catabolism in mammalian liver is shown in Figure 4-19. For practical purposes the reactions may be considered to be restricted to the cytosol. A so-called mitochondrial tyrosine transaminase has turned out to be identical with mitochondrial aspartate transaminase, its regulation having no direct relationship to the control of tyrosine metabolism.

Catabolism of tyrosine begins with a transamination, forming hydroxyphenylpyruvate, a step which is rate-limiting under usual conditions. The keto acid is then attacked by an hydroxylase, which simultaneously oxidizes the aromatic ring, decarboxylates the side chain, and moves the latter to an adjacent carbon atom on the ring. The product, homogentisate, is cleaved by an oxygenase to maleylacetoacetate, which, after isomerization to fumarylacetoacetate, is hydrolyzed to fumarate and acetoacetate. With such products, it is apparent why tyrosine (and phenylalanine) behaves as either a glucogenic or a ketogenic amino acid in various test systems. In any case, in yielding such useful metabolic fuels, this pathway is certainly ergogenic. None of the reactions other than the transamination is reversible.

With respect to its regulatory properties, mammalian tyrosine transaminase probably is the most intensively investigated enzyme in the current biochemical literature, resulting in the accumulation of a vast number of publications. Accordingly, it will be most convenient to discuss its regulation in general terms first, followed by a more detailed consideration of certain specific regulators, pointing out some of the current controversies as regards sites and mechanisms of action.

Tyrosine transaminase is induced by administration of a rather large number of substances, most of which have been demonstrated to function indirectly, by way of the adrenals, since their effectiveness is eliminated by adrenalectomy. Tyrosine, a substrate, often is included in this category. However, tyrosine is a direct (but slow-acting) inducer in adrenalectomized *young* rats (45 to 56 days) and, if accompanied by a minimal amount of glucocorticoid hormone for its permissive effects, seems to retain some efficacy even in adrenalectomized older rats. It may be that tyrosine transaminase, as it arises in the developing organism, is

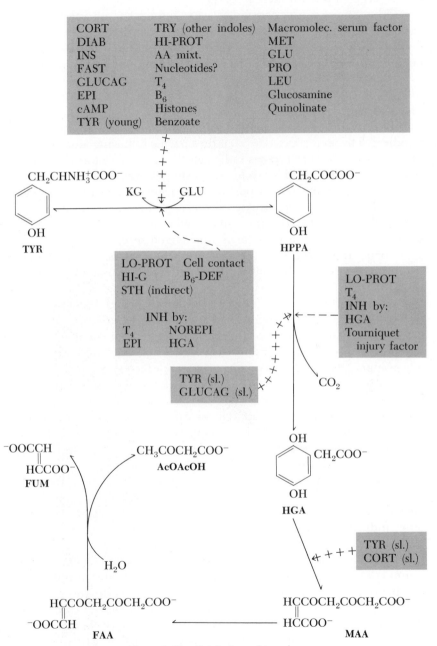

Figure 4–19. Catabolism of tyrosine.

just as substrate-inducible as tryptophan pyrrolase, but that this property is largely lost with increasing age.

Other amino acids reported to act as inducers in one or another of various test systems include tryptophan (and certain other indolic compounds such as 5-hydroxytryptophan and serotonin), methionine, glutamate, proline, and leucine. It has been shown that tryptophan derivatives become functional inducers only after decarboxylation to indoleamines. Administration of a casein hydrolysate and a high-protein diet also are effective.

That tyrosine transaminase is subject to a type of cofactor-induction is indicated by an increased level of the enzyme following administration of pyridoxine. Earlier reports indicated that the effect was inhibited by puromycin, not by actinomycin, suggesting a translational or at least post-transcriptional site and possibly a close analogy to the cofactor induction of tryptophan pyrrolase. However, later work gives no support to the notion that the cofactor stabilizes the transaminase, since the rate of degradation of the enzyme is unchanged after administration of pyridoxine. It is also claimed that the induction is blocked by actinomycin. Until these contradictions are resolved, conclusions as to mechanism would be premature.

By as yet unknown mechanisms, but not involving the adrenals, the transaminase is induced by certain nucleotides, histones, and certain organic acids such as benzoate and quinolinate (a metabolite of tryptophan). The enzyme is induced in some types of cultured cells by glucosamine and by a macromolecular serum factor.

Tyrosine transaminase is increased in level in the liver of animals made experimentally diabetic, and after the administration of several hormones, including thyroxine, glucocorticoids, insulin, glucagon (and fasting, which probably functions via increased secretion of glucagon), and epinephrine, the last two hormones utilizing cAMP as second messenger. All available evidence indicates that insulin, glucocorticoids, and the cAMP-utilizing hormones operate via separate and independent mechanisms, and possibly at separate and independent sites. Additional details concerning the actions of these hormones as well as of certain other inducers will be presented in a later section.

The tyrosine transaminase of adult rat liver exists in the form of four isoenzymes separable by hydroxylapatite column chromatography (numbered I to IV in order of elution). Type I is found also in kidney and heart and remains unchanged when regulatory influences alter the proportions of types II, III, and IV in liver. Formation of type II is induced by birth; its production undergoes a relative decline at 14 days after birth. Type IV appears first at weaning. A high-protein diet induces the formation of types II, III, and IV; glucocorticoid or glucagon induces mostly type II with some increase in type III; cAMP or epinephrine induces type II, and insulin type IV. In the diabetic rat type II predominates and type IV almost disappears.

Levels of the transaminase are decreased on low-protein or high-glucose diets, in pyridoxine deficiency, and by contact-inhibition among cells in culture. Administration of growth hormone to the adrenalectomized rat represses tyrosine transaminase and opposes its induction by glucocorticoids, but the effect is indirect, since it is not seen in the isolated perfused liver. By whatever mechanism growth hormone functions, however, its final effects appear to endure for some time, since liver slices from hypophysectomized rats are susceptible to glucocorticoid induction of the transaminase *in vitro*, whereas this ability is repressed in slices from normal rats. Although thyroxine and the catecholamines have been mentioned as inducers, both classes of hormones inhibit the action of the transaminase *in vitro*, as does homogentisate, a later metabolite in the catabolic pathway of tyrosine (possible negative feedback?).

Figure 4-20 depicts, in greater detail, the actions and proposed mechanisms of action of a selected group of regulatory agents upon induction and repression of tyrosine transaminase. It will be noted that there is considerable similarity to the regulatory array around tryptophan pyrrolase.

Substrate induction is shown as operating via a protective, antidegradative mechanism, more by analogy with the tryptophan system than by direct evidence. Pyridoxine (vitamin B_6) is presented as precursor of the transaminase coenzyme, but no mechanism is given for its inductive effect, since, as mentioned earlier, there is now no consensus on this. Induction by tryptophan usually is assumed to occur at the ribosomal level, as discussed earlier in this monograph; however, the effect is reported to be blocked by actinomycin.

A peculiar and as yet unexplained characteristic of tyrosine transaminase is its induction by the generally antigluconeogenic hormone, insulin, as well as by glucagon, catecholamines, and glucocorticoids. This effect, which is seen in the adrenalectomized rat, perfused liver, and in several types of hepatoma cells in culture, is particularly difficult to explain, since insulin is known to cause a decrease in the level of cAMP in liver, in contrast to the increase caused by glucagon and catecholamines. Since glucocorticoid induction is independent of cAMP altogether, it is probable that at least three distinct hormonal inductive mechanisms exist for this transaminase.

Although Figure 4-20 shows insulin and glucocorticoids acting at the level of transcription, and glucagon (as well as other cAMP-producers) operating between transcription and translation, this choice of sites is completely arbitrary. Evidence and opinions can be cited from the literature purporting to demonstrate that any one of these hormones may, in specific systems, be functioning at either pole of the nuclear-ribosomal axis.

In addition, the controversy concerning superinduction by actinomycin, discussed earlier in connection with tryptophan pyrrolase, exists also in relation to tyrosine transaminase. Here again, one school of

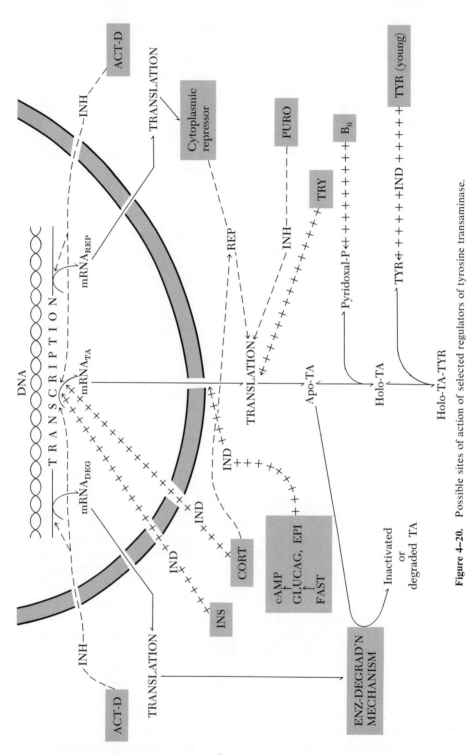

Figure 4-20. Possible sites of action of selected regulators of tyrosine transaminase.

thought contends that, under specified conditions, actinomycin inhibits transcription of an RNA messenger for synthesis of a degradative protein, whereas others find the most likely explanation to be blockage of synthesis of a labile cytoplasmic repressor protein (recent reports from the same laboratory contain the suggestion that the repressor may be a labile species of RNA). Glucocorticoid induction is then interpreted by the two sides, respectively, as occurring either at the site of transcription or via blockage of the repressor.

The question of the functional significance of the regulatory mechanisms just discussed for tyrosine transaminase may be raised, as it was for tryptophan pyrrolase. Again, experiments utilizing labeled substrate and intact rats or perfused liver show that the rate of oxidation of tyrosine to CO_2 is more sensitive to the supply of amino acid than to the administration of various inducing agents, despite the fact that the latter do effect an increase in the amount of enzyme in the liver. And again, as in the case of the pyrrolase, it may be suggested that supply of substrate may be the primary rate-controlling factor in this metabolic pathway also, with endocrine and other influences serving as secondary or back-up reserves.

There is evidence of regulation of enzyme steps subsequent to the transaminase. As can be seen in Figure 4-19, hydroxyphenylpyruvate hydroxylase is induced slightly by tyrosine or glucagon, its *activity* is inhibited by homogentisate and by a macromolecular factor released by tourniquet injury, and its synthesis repressed by thyroid hormones and a low-protein diet. Homogentisate oxygenase is induced by tyrosine and glucocorticoids, but both effects are slight.

Studies of temporal regulation of tyrosine transaminase are numerous. In several mammalian species, the enzyme has been shown to be included in the neonatal developmental group, the natural stimulus for its rise at that time being postnatal hypoglycemia and the consequent stimulation of secretion of glucagon. (It should be noted that the steep rise in hepatic tyrosine transaminase level usually observed during the first 12 hours after birth of the rat is ascribed by some to the separation of the newborn rats from their mothers in most laboratories.) Although administration of glucocorticoids to the near-term rat fetus does not induce appearance of the transaminase unless continued for a relatively long time, the enzyme is readily induced in the late rat fetus by glucagon, epinephrine, or cAMP. Birth sensitizes the enzyme-evoking mechanism to glucocorticoids. Development of the isoenzymic forms has been mentioned previously. The neonatal development of the transaminase in rats is blocked by adrenalectomy, actinomycin, and cycloheximide.

Explants of fetal rat liver in organ culture, if taken from the eighteenth gestational day to term, are amenable to premature induction of the transaminase by glucocorticoid, glucagon, or insulin. At the thirteenth day, glucocorticoid is not effective, but a combination of glucagon and cAMP is. Glucocorticoid induces the enzyme from the fourteenth or fifteenth day on. Explants of human fetal liver from the fourteenth to the twenty-fourth week of gestation exhibit no effects from glucocorticoid, glucagon, or insulin, but 26-week explants are inducible by glucocorticoid.

During the first 24 hours after birth of the rat, enzymes catalyzing steps after the transaminase also undergo characteristic alterations. Hydroxyphenylpyruvate hydroxylase and homogentisate oxygenase appear to trace out parallel increases and decreases in level, whereas fumarylacetoacetate hydrolase begins at a very high level, increases even farther for an hour or so, then drops abruptly.

Various investigators have estimated the half-life of the mRNA of tyrosine transaminase as 30 to 45 minutes in adult rat liver, and for the enzyme itself, 1.5 to 3 hours.

During the cell cycle in cultured hepatoma cells, tyrosine transaminase is inducible by glucocorticoids in the latter two-thirds of the postmitotic (G1) phase and the DNA synthesis (S) phase, but is noninducible in the premitotic (G2), mitotic (M), and first third of the postmitotic (G1) phases. During the noninducible phases, the enzyme is still synthesized from previously accumulated mRNA.

In senescent rats, various inductive mechanisms for tyrosine transaminase function more slowly than in younger animals.

Tyrosine transaminase levels in rats exhibit a seasonal cycle, being higher in winter and lower in summer. Adrenalectomy eliminates the winter rise.

Even more striking is the circadian rhythm, which results in as much as a fourfold difference in transaminase level in the course of 24 hours. The liver of the neonatal rat already shows evidence of a rhythm a few days after birth, although opposite in phase to the adult rhythm. Various endocrine factors have been proposed as driving forces in the tyrosine transaminase rhythm (glucocorticoids, catecholamines, pituitary, and pancreatic hormones), but the rhythm has been found to persist after excision of each of the glands of origin of the hormones. Neural control also has been postulated, but its primacy in this regard remains to be demonstrated. The circadian rhythm is said to be influenced in a positive direction by vagal-cholinergic stimulation, and in a negative direction by adrenergic stimulation and the resulting inhibitory influence of catecholamines upon the transaminase. It is probable that endocrine and neural factors serve to modulate whatever basic mechanism provides the primary drive.

In the rat, the variable most closely correlated with the rhythmic changes in level of hepatic tyrosine transaminase appears to be the timing of periods of maximum food intake. Being a nocturnal feeder, the rat attains maximum enzyme level at night, and hence exhibits a circadian rhythm which appears to be synchronous with the lighting cycle. Experiments have shown, however, that it is the intake of food and not the cycle of illumination which is the deciding factor. In fact, the closest approximation to an immediate cause of the cycle is the tryptophan content of the food, probably functioning by way of the potent control which tryptophan seems to have upon the level of polyribosomes in the liver cell. The "out-of-phase" cycle of the newborn rat has been explained by the probable daytime maximum food intake, when the mother is less active in her own feeding cycle.

A circadian rhythm is shown also by hydroxyphenylpyruvate hydroxylase (but not by homogentisate oxygenase), paralleling that of the transaminase but smaller in amplitude.

SUMMARY OF REGULATIONS OF INDIVIDUAL AMINO ACID PATHWAYS

Table 4-1 lists the effects of the major dietary and endocrine regulatory factors on whatever reaction of an amino acid's catabolic pathway has been shown to be rate-limiting. In the absence of specific information, an arbitrary choice has been made of a reaction which seemed most likely to be the controlling step in an ergogenic metabolic route. Threonine is omitted, since its major catabolic pathways are initiated by enzymes which are identical with serine dehydratase and serine-glycine transhy-

Table 4–1.   *Effects of Nutritional and Endocrine Factors on Rate-limiting Catabolic Reactions of Amino Acids*

AA	ENZ	CORT	GLUCAG, EPI, CAMP	FAST	DIAB	HI-PROT	HI-G	INS	STH	LO-PROT
ALA	GPT	+	+	+	+	+	−		−	−
CYS	Cystathionase	+ (sl., ♂)	+	− (sl.)		+	−			−
SER	Dehydratase	+	+	+	+	+	−	−	−	−
GLY	Transhydroxy-methylase	+		+	+				−	
ASP/										
GLU	GOT	+	+	+	+	+	−		−	
GLU	GDH	+		+	+ (sl.)	−		− ?		
ARG	LIV ORN-TA	+−	+	−	+	+	−	0	−	−
HIS	Histidase	+	+	+−	+	+	−	0	−	−
PRO	LIV Oxidase	+								−
MET	Cystathionine-synthase	+	+	−	+	+				−
BR-CH	KID Gen'l TA	+			+	+?				−
LYS	LYS-KG Reductase	+	+			+				
TRY	Pyrrolase	+	0 or −	+−	+	+	−		−	
PHE	Hydroxylase	+		−						−
TYR	TA	+	+	+	+	+	−		+	− (indirect) −

droxymethylase. In the cases of cysteine and methionine, cystathionase and cystathionine synthase have been assigned in that order; the two amino acids probably share a common ergogenic pathway, and both enzymes are subject to very similar regulation in any event.

If the relatively few exceptions are ignored temporarily, then the general picture becomes obvious. The controlling step in the conversion of most amino acids to ergogenic fragments is an enzyme which is induced by one or more of these factors: glucocorticoids, catecholamines-glucagon-cAMP, fasting, diabetes, and high-protein diet; and repressed by one or more of these factors: high-glucose diet, insulin, growth hormone, and low-protein diet. It also is obvious that there is no purely gluconeogenic regulatory drive. The same array of regulators appears, whether an amino acid belongs to the glucogenic, combined glucogenic-ketogenic, or purely ketogenic camp, all of which reinforces the thesis of this monograph, that the biological value of these regulatory systems resides in the acceleration, on demand, of pathways producing energy-yielding fragments, with the additional formation of glucose as a most useful by-product.

Some of the exceptions and oddities in the table are as interesting as the general picture. The lack of inductive effect by glucagon on tryptophan pyrrolase, the failure of STH to repress tyrosine transaminase directly in the liver, and the induction of the latter enzyme by insulin (as well as in the diabetic!) all are anomalies which defy explanation at this time. The variable and, in several cases, negative effect of fasting deserves some attention. The abnormal response to fasting seems to be restricted to essential amino acids, suggesting that, in the course of evolution, it has proved advantageous to conserve essential amino acids in at least this one condition out of the several which customarily lead to increased rates of catabolism of the amino acids.

REFERENCES

Deamination and Related Pathways of Metabolism:
Regulation in the Adult

Knox, W. E., Auerbach, V. H., and Lin, E. C. C.: Enzymatic and metabolic adaptations in animals. Physiol. Rev. *36*:164–254 (1956).
Knox, W. E., and Greengard, O.: The regulation of some enzymes of nitrogen metabolism—an introduction to enzyme physiology. Adv. Enz. Reg. *3*:247–313 (1965).
Kenney, F. T.: Hormonal regulation of synthesis of liver enzymes. *In:* Munro, H. N. (ed.): Mammalian Protein Metabolism. Vol. 4. New York, Academic Press, Inc., 1970, pp. 131–176.
Kaplan, J. H., and Pitot, H. C.: The regulation of intermediary amino acid metabolism in animal tissues. *In:* Munro, H. N. (ed.): Mammalian Protein Metabolism. Vol. 4. New York, Academic Press, Inc., 1970, pp. 387–443.
Rosen, F., and Milholland, R. J.,: Control of enzyme activity by glucocorticoids. *In:* Rechcigl, M., Jr. (ed.): Enzyme Synthesis and Degradation in Mammalian Systems. Baltimore, University Park Press, 1971, pp. 77–102.

Freedland, R. A., and Szepesi, B.: Control of enzyme activity: nutritional factors. *In*: Rechcigl, M., Jr. (ed.): Enzyme Synthesis and Degradation in Mammalian Systems. Baltimore, University Park Press, 1971, pp. 103–140.
Gelehrter, T. D.: Regulatory mechanisms of enzyme synthesis: enzyme induction. *In*: Rechcigl, M., Jr. (ed.): Enzyme Synthesis and Degradation in Mammalian Systems. Baltimore, University Park Press, 1971, pp. 165–199.
Pitot, H. C., Kaplan, J., and Čihák, A.: Translational regulation of enzyme levels in liver. *In*: Rechcigl, M., Jr. (ed.): Enzyme Synthesis and Degradation in Mammalian Systems. Baltimore, University Park Press, 1971, pp. 216–235.
Rechcigl, M., Jr.: Intracellular protein turnover and the roles of synthesis and degradation in regulation of enzyme levels. *In*: Rechcigl, M., Jr. (ed.): Enzyme Synthesis and Degradation in Mammalian Systems. Baltimore, University Park Press, 1971, pp. 236–310.
Pitot, H. C., and Yatvin, M. B: Interrelationships of mammalian hormones and enzyme levels in vivo. Physiol. Rev. *53*:228–325 (1973).

Developmental Regulation

Herrmann, H., and Tootle, M. A.: Specific and general aspects of the development of enzymes and metabolic pathways. Physiol. Rev. *44*:289–371 (1964).
Greengard, O.: The developmental formation of enzymes in rat liver. *In*: Litwack, G. (ed.): Biochemical Actions of Hormones, Vol. 1. New York, Academic Press, Inc., 1970, pp. 53–87.
Moog, F: The control of enzyme activity in mammals in early development and in old age. *In*: Rechcigl, M., Jr. (ed.): Enzyme Synthesis and Degradation in Mammalian Systems. Baltimore, University Park Press, 1971, pp. 47–76.
Räihä, N. C. R.: The development of some enzymes of aminoacid metabolism in the human liver. *In*: Jonxis, J. H. P., Visser, H. K. A., and Troelstra, J. A. (eds.): Metabolic Processes in the Foetus and Newborn Infant. Baltimore, The Williams & Wilkins Company, 1971, pp. 26–34.
Sereni, F., and Principi, N.: The regulation of liver function during development. *In*: Benson, P. (ed.): The Biochemistry of Development. London, Spastics International Medical Publications, 1971, pp. 1–13.
Knox, W. E.: Enzyme Patterns in Fetal, Adult, and Neoplastic Rat Tissues. Basel, S. Karger, 1972.

Rhythmic Regulation

Wurtman, R. J.: Diurnal rhythms in mammalian protein metabolism. *In*: Munro, H. N. (ed.): Mammalian Protein Metabolism. Vol. 4. New York, Academic Press, Inc., 1970, pp. 445–479.
Fuller, R. W.: Rhythmic changes in enzyme activity and their control. *In*: Rechcigl, M., Jr. (ed.): Enzyme Synthesis and Degradation in Mammalian Systems. Baltimore, University Park Press, 1971, pp. 311–338.

5

DEAMINATION, GLUCONEOGENESIS, AND RELATED PATHWAYS. PART II: DISPOSAL OF NITROGEN

INTRODUCTION

As indicated at various points in this monograph, the ammonia which arrives in the liver through the portal blood, as well as that which arises as the result of deamination reactions within the liver, undergoes detoxication chiefly by conversion to urea through the ornithine cycle. To a lesser extent, the liver synthesizes glutamine from ammonia and exports it to other tissues for disposal. In kidney, glutamine from liver is hydrolyzed to liberate ammonia, which, along with ammonia derived from renal deamination of amino acids, plays an important role in acid-base balance.

The total 24-hour excretion of urinary urea plus ammonia varies with the state of nitrogen balance and dietary nitrogen intake, the urea component predominating by a wide margin under ordinary conditions.

However, the proportion of total urinary nitrogen represented by free ammonia varies with the state of acid-base balance. In extreme acidosis, ammonia can predominate and urea can be reduced to a subordinate status.

Chapter 4 delineated the regulatory mechanisms concerned with the deamination processes and with the pathways of disposal of the resultant carbon skeletons. Since nature tends to "cover all bets," it might be anticipated that the disposal pathways for waste ammonia also are under regulation. As will be seen in the subsequent sections of this chapter, the chief pathway, the ornithine cycle, is regulated in the manner which we have come to expect of ergogenic catabolic routes, whereas the glutamine pathway, although not entirely refractory to these same factors, is controlled largely by the exigencies of acid-base balance.

ORNITHINE CYCLE

Characteristics of the Cycle

Figure 5–1 pictures the reactions of the ornithine cycle, the ancillary ornithine transaminase reaction, the intracellular location of each enzyme, and some indication of the rate of each reaction in adult rat liver.

The reactions of the cycle begin with carbamyl phosphate synthetase (The Enzyme Commission favors the spelling "carbamoyl"), which catalyzes condensation of a molecule each of ammonia, carbon dioxide, and phosphate, with the sacrifice of two molecules of ATP. Although carbamyl phosphate also is a precursor of pyrimidines, its synthesis for that purpose is catalyzed by a glutamine-utilizing cytoplasmic enzyme which has no specific connection with the ornithine cycle.

Carbamyl phosphate synthetase is activated allosterically by N-acetyl-glutamate. The activator is synthesized from acetyl-CoA and glutamate by an intramitochondrial transacetylase which is strongly activated by arginine. Since arginine is the penultimate product of the cycle, we have here an unusual example of positive feedback, the physiological significance of which is unknown at this time.

The carbamyl moiety is transferred to ornithine to form citrulline by ornithine transcarbamylase. The incipient urea molecule then receives its second nitrogen atom from the alpha-amino group of aspartate, which condenses with citrulline in the argininosuccinate synthetase reaction, consuming another molecule of ATP. In the argininosuccinate lyase (argininosuccinase) reaction, the carbon chain of aspartate leaves in the guise of fumarate, forming arginine. (The synthetase and lyase together sometimes are referred to in the literature as arginine synthetase or the arginine-synthesizing system, since the combined activities of

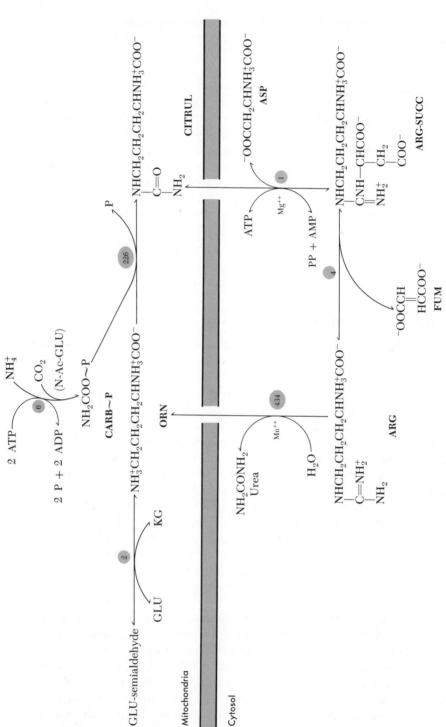

Figure 5–1. Reactions of ornithine cycle, including intracellular location and specific activities (numbers adjacent to reaction arrows) based upon values rounded off to nearest whole number from Knox, W. E.: Enzyme Patterns in Fetal, Adult and Neoplastic Rat Tissues. Basel.

the two enzymes occasionally are assayed as a unit.) The cycle terminates with the hydrolysis of arginine, catalyzed by arginase, yielding urea and re-forming a molecule of ornithine to continue the cycle.

The energy requirements for urea synthesis are of some interest. Although utilization of three molecules of ATP in order to synthesize one molecule of a waste product would appear to be rather profligate on the part of the liver cell, even granting the necessity of disposing of the highly toxic ammonia molecule, closer examination indicates that the cycle actually functions with little expenditure of energy. Fumarate liberated from the cycle in the lyase reaction is converted to malate, which is then oxidized to oxaloacetate. The glutamate-oxaloacetate transaminase reaction then not only converts oxaloacetate to aspartate, thus providing this compound for the cycle, but also furnishes a route for entry of the amino groups of most amino acids into the cycle, via individual transaminations with ketoglutarate. The oxidation of malate to oxaloacetate, coupled to the mechanisms for oxidative phosphorylation, can generate the equivalent of three high-energy bonds, thus making the entire cycle self-supporting.

It will be noted in Figure 5–1 that the first two reactions of the cycle and ornithine transaminase are mitochondrial, whereas the last three reactions occur in the cytosol. Consequently, continued operation of the cycle requires a steady flow of ornithine into and citrulline out of the mitochondria. In addition, the conversion of fumarate to oxaloacetate requires mitochondrial uptake of the former (or its hydrated product, malate) and formation of the latter; intramitochondrial transamination then occurs, with release of aspartate. There is no information available on the possible role played by these transport processes in the regulation of the ornithine cycle.

Figure 5–1 indicates the specific activities of the enzymes of the cycle (plus ornithine transaminase) in the liver of the adult rat. Keeping in mind the possibility that, *in vivo*, enzymes may not be operating at their optimum rates as assayed *in vitro*, nevertheless the argininosuccinate synthetase step appears to be rate-limiting for the cycle, followed closely by the lyase. Consequently, special attention must be accorded these two enzymes in considering the physiological significance of reported regulatory responses. It is an interesting commentary upon fashions in research to note how much effort has been and still is being expended on investigation of the regulation of the arginase reaction, in view of the probability that nothing short of a hepatic catastrophe could bring the level of arginase down to the critical range.

Although the specific activity of ornithine transaminase seems to be as low as that of the rate-limiting reaction(s) of the cycle proper, the functional relation of this transaminase to the cycle is not at all certain (see following discussion).

Role of Ornithine Transaminase

Many of the characteristics of the hepatic (as well as renal) enzyme have been discussed in connection with arginine metabolism in the preceding chapter. Instead of repeating the details of that discussion, the various regulatory influences upon this enzyme are listed in Figure 5–2, along with those affecting the enzymes of the ornithine cycle proper. It will be noted that, aside from certain peculiarities not shared with the cycle (e.g., the influences of ornithine and some other amino acids, estrogens, and branched-chain amino acids, and the equivocal effects of glucocorticoids), ornithine transaminase is regulated in the main by the usual gluconeogenic factors.

Although it has been suggested that this enzyme subserves an anaplerotic function, supplying or removing ornithine from the cycle at rate-limiting speed, this seems highly unlikely. There is no evidence that ornithine is ever in short supply in the liver. Indeed, given the plentiful quantities of arginine and the enormous activity of arginase, it is difficult to imagine circumstances in which the transaminase could exert a regulatory function on the cycle. It is more likely that the chief physiological role of ornithine transaminase in liver is that of a controlling step in the catabolism of arginine, a role which would require the enzyme to be subject to much the same type of regulation as that affecting the ornithine cycle.

Positive Regulators of the Cycle

There have been many observations over the years to the effect that the usual factors or conditions predisposing the organism toward gluconeogenesis (or ergoneogenesis) result, in either the intact animal or the perfused liver, in augmentation of the rate of synthesis of urea. As can be seen in Figure 5–2, these data are readily explicable in terms of direct effects of the regulatory factors upon one or more enzymes of the cycle, particularly those which are probably rate-limiting *in vivo*.

All five enzymes of the cycle are increased in level in the liver by a high-protein diet, fasting, or administration of glucocorticoids. (*Prolonged* fasting in man results in eventual decrease in urea output to rather low levels, probably a consequence of the drastically reduced supply of plasma amino acids, particularly alanine, coming from the muscle mass in these circumstances. The higher levels of the enzymes of the ornithine cycle induced by fasting may be physiologically useful only in the early stages of the fast.) In the alloxan-diabetic or glucagon-treated rat, only the three slowest enzymes (carbamyl phosphate synthetase, argininosuccinate synthetase, and lyase) are induced. Thyroid hormones induce the synthesis of either or both of the arginine-synthetase enzymes as well as of arginase.

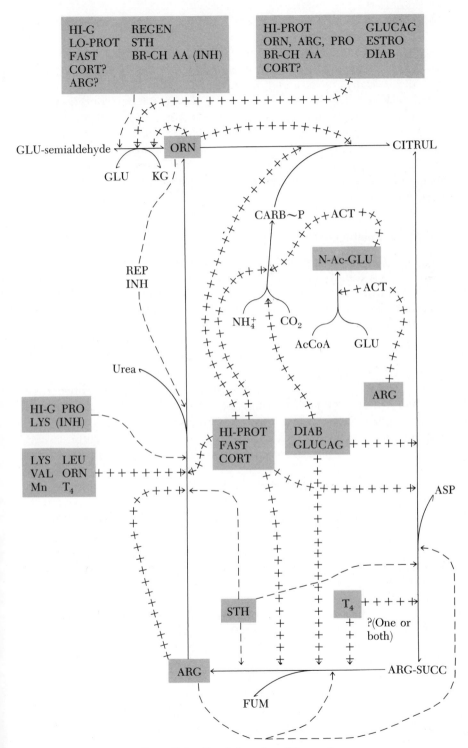

Figure 5-2. Regulation of ornithine cycle.

Several substances of low molecular weight also influence the cycle in a positive direction. Carbamyl phosphate synthetase is activated, probably allosterically, by N-acetylglutamate. Rat liver ornithine transcarbamylase is induced by ornithine under certain dietary conditions. In various types of mammalian cell cultures arginase is induced by the presence of arginine, ornithine, lysine, leucine, and valine. Under similar conditions manganese induces arginase by stabilizing the enzyme. A curious effect is seen in animals on arginine-free diets: arginase remains unchanged in activity, while all other enzymes of the cycle increase in level significantly.

Negative Regulators of the Cycle

As might be anticipated, lack of certain positive factors has a repressive effect on the cycle, e.g., low-protein diet and adrenalectomy. For some unknown reason the latter operation depresses the level of arginase much more drastically than that of the other enzymes of the cycle.

One of the reasons accounting for the popularity of arginase as an experimental object is the discovery that much of its regulation is exerted through alterations in its rate of degradation. Under normal conditions, the rates of synthesis and degradation of this enzyme are equal, as they are for any substance which exists in a steady state of concentration. In fasting, the rate of synthesis remains relatively constant, but the rate of degradation falls to zero. On shifting from a high- to a low-protein diet, the rate of degradation increases, and that of synthesis decreases. Findings of this sort have strengthened the belief that, in mammalian organisms (in contrast to bacteria), induction can be effected as readily through decreased degradation as through increased synthesis.

Of the usual antiglucogenic endocrine factors, growth hormone (STH) represses argininosuccinate synthetase and lyase as well as arginase. The effects of insulin, on the other hand, are completely obscure. Although the three slowest enzymes of the cycle are elevated in level in the alloxan-diabetic rat, administration of insulin to such an animal results first in an increase in the rate-limiting enzymes (plus arginase), followed by a decrease to the diabetic values. It has been suggested that the effects of diabetes on the ornithine cycle are due, not to an absolute deficiency of insulin, but to an unopposed surplus of glucagon, its hormonal antagonist in many situations.

In mammalian cell cultures, the presence of arginine represses synthesis of argininosuccinate synthetase and lyase, whereas the synthesis of arginase is repressed by ornithine, proline, and glucose. Lysine and ornithine inhibit arginase activity *in vitro*, cases of competitive inhibition through structural similarity.

Administration of tryptophan to man inhibits gluconeogenesis and urea production, probably through formation of quinolinate, a tryptophan metabolite which is known to suppress gluconeogenesis.

Temporal Regulation

In the human fetus the activities of carbamyl phosphate synthetase, ornithine transcarbamylase, argininosuccinate lyase, and arginase are measurable from the fiftieth day of gestation. Peaks in activity are seen on the sixtieth and ninetieth days, except for the transcarbamylase, which lacks the second peak. All enzymes measured except arginase reach adult values before birth.

There is general agreement that the ornithine cycle enzymes of rat liver begin to develop in the late fetal period, reach their first peak early in neonatal life, then exhibit a second spurt of development at about the time of weaning. More detailed study of arginase reveals that the earlier peak is enhanced by thyroxine (not by glucocorticoids) and the later peak by glucocorticoids (not by thyroxine), which can raise the level of enzyme to adult values in 24 hours if administered on the fifth to the eighth postnatal day. The second peak is obliterated by adrenalectomy on the twelfth day. These and related observations indicate clearly the specificity of developmental inducers on the temporal scale.

A developmental study of the arginine synthetase system in the rat (probably reflecting the properties of the rate-limiting argininosuccinate synthetase) confirms the spurt in level of the enzyme(s) during the first few days after birth. Although the inducers tested have no effect on the fetus, glucocorticoid induces the system in the 1-day-old rat and glucagon does the same in the 5-day-old rat. In contrast to the fetus *in vivo*, explants of near-term fetuses in organ culture are amenable to induction of this enzyme system by glucocorticoid, glucagon, and cAMP.

The developmental pattern of the enzymes of the ornithine cycle meets the requirements of mammals, which, as ureotelic organisms, must provide their own urea-synthesizing machinery once they depart the maternal environment and its system for disposal of waste ammonia.

GLUTAMINE PATHWAY

Introduction*

The kidney reacts to acidosis and alkalosis in a number of ways, not all of which are understood at this time. In addition to the phenomena

---

*Only a bare minimum of information concerning the role of the kidney in acid-base balance will be included in this section; this will be sufficient for the purpose at hand. Detailed discussions may be found in the monograph of this series, *Acid-Base Regulation: Its Physiology and Pathophysiology*, or in textbooks of biochemistry or physiology.

related to ammonia metabolism which will be discussed shortly, the kidney of the acidotic animal exhibits an increase in the activity of the hexose monophosphate shunt (or pentose) pathway, and hypertrophy characterized by increased levels of RNA and protein. The hypertrophy resembles, but is causally distinct from, the compensatory hypertrophy following unilateral nephrectomy. In alkalosis, various species of experimental animals and man excrete in the urine increased amounts of organic acid anions such as citrate and ketoglutarate. It has been found that high concentrations of bicarbonate increase the rate of efflux (or decrease the rate of influx) of citrate from rabbit kidney mitochondria, thus possibly accounting for the increased clearance of citrate in alkalosis.

One of the two ways in which the kidney helps to preserve acid-base balance in the face of an acid load is the excretion of an acid urine. Beginning with a glomerular filtrate at pH 7.4, kidney tubule cells are able to exchange hydrogen ions for sodium ions in the lumen of the tubule to the extent of depressing the pH of the urine to a minimal value of about 4.4. Thus, unwanted acid is removed from the organism and valuable cations such as sodium are retained.

Since a minimal pH of 4.4 in the urine severely limits the amount of hydrogen ion which can be eliminated by the acidification mechanism, another renal device for excretion of acid has evolved, which, in fact, has much greater capacity than the cation exchange pathway. Ammonia, a base, is produced within the kidney tubule cells and diffuses out into the lumen, where it can combine with hydrogen ions to form the weak acid, NH_4^+. At the pH of urine, the ammonium ion is largely undissociated. Hence, a means is made available for the carriage of hydrogen ions without undue depression of pH. It is this second renal mechanism for the excretion of acid which will be the subject of the subsequent discussion.

Role of Liver in the Glutamine Pathway

As can be seen in Figure 5–3, nitrogenous raw materials come to the liver via the portal blood in the form of amino acids, glutamine, and free ammonia (ammonium ions). For the sake of simplicity the arterial supply of the liver is omitted; this influx of blood supplies much the same types of substances, except that free ammonia is present only in traces.

Portal ammonia joins the intracellular ammonia pool, most of which is drawn upon for the synthesis of urea. The pool is supplied also with ammonia from the deamination of amino acids, and, to a slight extent, from hydrolysis of glutamine (via hepatic glutaminases). The liver generally synthesizes more glutamine than it hydrolyzes; virtually all of the ammonia not directed into the ornithine cycle eventuates in this amide. The glutamine thus produced, urea, and amino acids not deaminated or

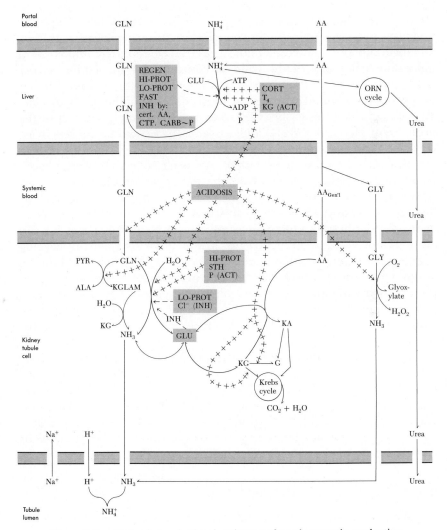

Figure 5-3. Glutamine and related pathways of renal ammonia production.

required for other purposes by the liver are all exported into the systemic blood.

Although glutamine synthetase in various types of mammalian cells in culture is repressed by glutamine, there is no evidence for this mechanism of control in normal liver. The enzyme is induced in young rats by glucocorticoid and thyroid hormones and is repressed by low-protein diets, fasting, adrenalectomy, and in the residual regenerating liver, after partial hepatectomy. High-protein diets have been reported variously as decreasing or having no effect on the enzyme concentration. Of uncertain physiological significance are the reported inhibition of glutamine synthetase of the Chinese hamster liver by alanine, serine, ADP, phosphate, and CTP, and activation by ketoglutarate. Similar properties are exhibited by the rat liver enzyme: inhibition by glycine, alanine, beta-alanine, serine, CTP, and carbamyl phosphate, all in the presence of Mn^{++}, not Mg^{++}, and activation by ketoglutarate, less by citrate, and a slight amount by NAD.

In contrast to the above rather confusing collection of regulatory factors, and of greater interest from the standpoint of acid-base balance, is the reported increase in glutamine synthesis by the liver of the acidotic dog. Isolated rat liver, when perfused with blood at pH 7.15, shows decreased synthesis of glutamine compared with controls at pH 7.4, but even greater decrease in *consumption* of the amide, the net result being augmented output of glutamine by the liver. On the other hand, in the acidotic dog, the feedback signal to the liver appears to be the load of portal blood ammonia, which is significantly increased in acidosis. This increase may be due to the greater extraction of glutamine from arterial blood by the intestinal cells of the acidotic animal, followed by hydrolysis.

Hepatic glutamine synthetase in the rat belongs to the weaning developmental group of enzymes. The fetus contains low but detectable activity. At 10 days after birth, there is an abrupt rise in level until about day 22, after which the level remains steady. Adrenalectomy or administration of glucocorticoids or glutamine has no effect on the development, but it can be accelerated by thyroid hormones in the late fetus or early neonate.

Role of Kidney in the Glutamine Pathway

As can be seen in Figure 5-3, kidney takes up from the systemic blood glutamine, various amino acids, prominent among which is glycine, and urea, this last substance having no direct bearing on acid-base balance. A few individual amino acids actually are added to the blood by the kidney. The amount of glutamine extracted by the kidney is relatively large and increases in acidosis. The uptake of amino acids, even of glycine, is relatively small, and generally is reported to undergo no great changes in acidosis. These observations suggest that, whereas amino acids in general, and glycine in particular, may well contribute to the pool of ammonia, the *variable* component of that pool, which must increase and decrease with the state of acid-base balance, necessarily is provided by glutamine.

It is not known whether the increased extraction of glutamine by the kidney in acidosis is due to a direct effect of the acidotic condition on a transport mechanism for glutamine, or whether it is simply the result of increased intrarenal utilization of the compound, thus augmenting the rate of influx by mass action.

As may be inferred from the tone of the preceding discussion and from the preceding sideheadings, glutamine is regarded as the major source of urinary ammonia. However, it may be advantageous to mention briefly the few minor sources. About 20 years ago it was observed that kidney slices from chronically acidotic rats produce ammonia at an increased rate from glutamine, glycine, and leucine. Chronic alkalosis results in changes in the opposite direction. Neither condition causes alteration in ammonia production from aspartate or alanine. The last observation suggests that the general transaminase systems are unaffected by acidosis. Aside from the usually reported increase in glutamine hydrolysis, the remaining data point to a probable increased level in glycine oxidase (generally regarded now as identical with D-amino acid oxidase) and L-amino acid oxidase (for which leucine is an excellent substrate). Since glycine is, at best, a minor source of urinary ammonia, and since the L-amino acid oxidase is present in few biological sites in appreciable concentration outside the rat kidney, these two pathways have attracted little investigative interest in recent years and will not be pursued further here.

Although Figure 5-3 depicts the transdeamination pathway for amino acids in general, this is solely for the sake of completeness. There is no evidence that this pathway contributes a significant part of the readily *variable* output of ammonia which responds to alterations in the acid-base status of the organism.

One system which produces ammonia from glutamine, glutaminase II, or keto acid–activated glutaminase, is not a true glutaminase at all but consists of a system of two enzymes. The first is a glutamine–keto acid transaminase which removes the amino group of glutamine, producing ketoglutaramate. Removal of the amide group is then catalyzed by an amidase, which forms free ammonia in a purely hydrolytic reaction. Although this system (specifically, the transaminase component) increases in activity in acidosis, its low level in the kidney, as compared with other glutaminases, does not permit any major role in acid-base regulation.

Rat kidney, and probably that of other species, contains at least two types of "true" glutaminases. The minor component constitutes only 10 to 15 per cent of the total, is activated by organic acid anions such as maleate and N-acetylglutamate, is not activated by phosphate, and probably plays no significant role in acid-base regulation.

The phosphate-activated glutaminase (glutaminase I) of kidney accounts for most of the hydrolysis of glutamine which occurs in that organ, and plays a major part in renal ammonia production, particularly in the response to acidosis. The molecule of glutamate resulting from glutaminase action can yield yet another molecule of ammonia via the glutamate dehydrogenase reaction. Ammonia produced by these and other reactions in the kidney tubule cell diffuses outward in two directions, toward the blood and toward the tubule lumen, the partition depending upon the relative acidity of the two "sinks." Since the liquid in the lumen is acidified in acidosis, ammonia is automatically directed where needed. It is of interest that the phosphate-activated glutaminase and glutamate dehydrogenase both are located within the mitochondria. The residual carbon chain, ketoglutarate, may be channeled into the pathways of gluconeogenesis or may be oxidized to CO_2.

Although the phosphate-activated renal glutaminase is decreased in level by a low-protein diet and increased in level by a high-protein diet and by the administration of growth hormone, these instances of regulation appear to be related to fluctuations in protein metabolism in general, not to regulation of acid-base balance. Likewise, activation of the enzyme by phosphate and inhibition of this effect by chloride, both occurring in the physiological range of ion concentrations, seem also to be unrelated to acid-base balance, since no significant alterations in the intracellular concentrations of these ions occur in acidosis or alkalosis. On the other hand, inhibition of the activity of this glutaminase by physiological concentrations of glutamate may indeed be relevant to the problem at hand, as will be discussed shortly.

The history of investigation of the regulation of ammonia production in kidney is characterized by an unfortunate succession of promising hypotheses, each of which has met its demise following the accumulation of further factual information.

Early observations on the acidotic rat indicated an adaptive increase in renal glutaminase (probably type I) level in that condition, thus providing an apparently satisfactory explanation for the adaptive increase in ammonia excretion. However, comparison with the dog reveals that, in the latter species, the increased excretion of ammonia is not accompanied by alteration in the level of renal glutaminase. Furthermore, in the rat itself, blockage of induction of enzyme synthesis by administration of actinomycin D does not simultaneously block adaptive ammonia production.

A glutamine synthetase exists in rat kidney (also in rabbit and guinea pig), undergoing alterations in activity converse to those of glutaminase with changes in the acid-base status of the animal; unfortunately, the generality of this adaptive mechanism is destroyed by the absence of the synthetase from dog kidney.

Species differences underlie much of the difficulty in construction of a universally applicable hypothesis for the biochemical basis of adaptive ammonia production. Herbivores such as rabbits and guinea pigs, which normally excrete alkaline urine, respond to acidosis with only moderate elevation in output of ammonia, probably a reflection of their relatively low levels of renal glutaminase. Kidneys of omnivores, such as rat and dog, produce both ammonia and carbohydrate from glutamine and glutamate, whereas kidneys of herbivores form only free ammonia from glutamine and only carbohydrate from glutamate. In addition, within the group of omnivores, there exist distinct differences between rat and dog, some of which have been mentioned already, others of which will be noted subsequently.

A new line of investigation has been opened by the discovery mentioned previously that physiological concentrations of glutamate inhibit the *activity* of phosphate-activated renal glutaminase. The probable relevance of this discovery is strengthened by the fact that renal concentrations of glutamate are found to be depressed in acidosis and elevated in alkalosis.

Recent investigations have centered upon the mechanism whereby the acidotic condition results in a decrease in the concentration of glutamate. One such postulated mechanism has gone the way of the other unsuccessful hypotheses. Under certain conditions, in certain test systems, acidosis is found to be accompanied by an augmented rate of renal gluconeogenesis. An increase in the rate of gluconeogenesis from glutamate (via ketoglutarate) would lower the concentration of that inhibitor of the glutaminase reaction, thus allowing an increased rate of deamination of glutamine, and in addition would produce more ammonia by increased deamination of glutamate. Unfortunately, in some species, acidosis (and increased ammonia excretion) is not accompanied by an increase in renal gluconeogenesis. In kidney slices, inhibition of gluconeogenesis from glutamate or ketoglutarate (e.g., using malonate) does not inhibit the increased ammonia production of acidosis. Finally, it has been found that kidney mitochondria, which lack the enzymes for performance of gluconeogenesis, nevertheless increase their utilization of glutamine when exposed to a lower pH.

On a quantitative basis, disposal of the carbon chain of glutamate (ketoglutarate) by complete oxidation via the Krebs cycle mechanism in renal tissue exceeds the fraction disposed of by gluconeogenesis (by a factor of five or six in the dog). Some investigators believe that the rate-limiting factor in ammoniagenesis by kidney lies in the amount of available NAD(P), or in the NAD(P)/NAD(P)H ratio. Since glutamate dehydrogenase competes with other NAD(P)-requiring enzymes for the cofactor, the instantaneous concentration of glutamate in the mitochondria may be controlled by the load of oxidizable substrates present. Since ketoglutarate itself is one such substrate, the elements of a self-limiting negative feedback system are present. Of course, this scheme still leaves unanswered the primary question: What acidosis-generated signal or mechanism results in the augmented utilization of glutamate, or in the lessened load of oxidizable substrates?

Comparative and Developmental Aspects of the Kidney Pathways

In species normally excreting an acid urine there would appear to be little need for *renal* glutamine synthetase. Indeed, a survey of six mammalian species found this enzyme in the kidneys only of those animals excreting a neutral or alkaline urine. A direct relationship exists, on the other hand, between the level of renal glutaminase (and, to some extent, hepatic glutamine synthetase) and the normal urinary acidity of the species.

In rat kidney, the phosphate-activated glutaminase characteristic of that tissue is found in significant concentration in the late fetal period, then increases two- to threefold (paralleling the growth of the kidney) during the first 4 postnatal days. From the ninth to the twenty-first postnatal day, the glutaminase level rises more or less linearly from about one-third to about three-fourths the adult values. The phosphate-independent glutaminase is detectable in kidney just before birth and remains at a low level during the first postnatal week.

For purposes of comparison, in rat liver, in which the function of glutaminases was not emphasized in the preceding discussions, the characteristic kidney type of glutaminase is present in high concentration in the late fetal period, drops toward birth, and continues to decrease after birth, whereas the liver type of glutaminase begins its developmental spurt in the late fetus.

REFERENCES

Ornithine Cycle

Knox, W. E., and Greengard, O.: Regulation of some enzymes of nitrogen metabolism. Adv. Enz. Reg. *3*:282–291 (1965).

Kaplan, J. H., and Pitot, H. C.: Regulation of intermediary amino acid metabolism. *In:* Munro, H. N. (ed.): Mammalian Protein Metabolism. Vol. 4. New York, Academic Press, Inc., 1970, pp. 402–407.

Freedland, R. A., and Szepesi, B.: Control of enzyme activity: nutritional factors. *In:* Rechcigl, M., Jr. (ed.): Enzyme Synthesis and Degradation in Mammalian Systems. Baltimore, University Park Press, 1971, p. 110.

Rechcigl, M., Jr.: Intracellular protein turnover and the roles of synthesis and degradation in regulation of enzyme levels. *In:* Rechcigl, M., Jr. (ed.): Enzyme Synthesis and Degradation in Mammalian Systems. Baltimore, University Park Press, 1971, pp. 264–265.

Glutamine and Related Pathways

Knox, W. E., and Greengard, O.: Regulation of some enzymes of nitrogen metabolism. Adv. Enz. Reg. *3*:291–297 (1965).

Lotspeich, W. D.: Metabolic aspects of acid-base change. Science *155*:1066–1075 (1967).

Kaplan, J. H., and Pitot, H. C.: Regulation of intermediary amino acid metabolism. *In:* Munro, H. N. (ed.): Mammalian Protein Metabolism. Vol. 4. New York, Academic Press, Inc., 1970, pp. 421–422.

Cahill, G. F., Jr., and Owen, O. E.: The role of the kidney in the regulation of protein metabolism. *In:* Munro, H. N. (ed.): Mammalian Protein Metabolism. Vol. 4. New York, Academic Press, Inc., 1970, pp. 573–577.

Pitts, R. F.: The role of ammonia production and excretion in regulation of acid-base balance. New Engl. J. Med. *284*:32–38 (1971).

Developmental Aspects

Linder-Horowitz, M.: Changes in glutaminase activities of rat liver and kidney during pre- and post-natal development. Biochem. J. *114*:65–70 (1969).

Greengard, O.: The developmental formation of enzymes in rat liver. *In:* Litwack, G. (ed.): Biochemical Actions of Hormones. Vol. 1. New York, Academic Press, Inc., 1970, pp. 57–66.

Räihä, N. C. R.: Development of arginine and ornithine metabolism in the mammal. *In:* Benson, P. (ed.): The Biochemistry of Development. London, Spastics International Medical Publications, 1971, pp. 141–160.

6

NON-ERGOGENIC PATHWAYS OF AMINO ACID METABOLISM: SELECTED EXAMPLES

INTRODUCTION

Previous chapters have dealt with mass movements of metabolites and with those major metabolic pathways which are involved in production of energy for the maintenance and growth of the mammalian organism. There exist in addition, however, many specialized pathways of amino acid metabolism which appear to have no significance in ergogenesis, but rather are used for the formation of special products which have some value to the organism.

No attempt will be made to discuss all of the nonergogenic reactions of the amino acids, if for no other reason than that the regulatory aspects of many have not been investigated. Instead, a selected group of examples will be covered.

It has not been considered within the province of this monograph to cover the regulation of protein synthesis *per se*, although all discussions of induction or repression of enzymes certainly represent specialized examples of the general phenomenon. However, the synthesis of two nonenzyme proteins will be touched upon in this chapter in connection with the metabolism of certain amino acids (hemoglobin in the case of glycine, and collagen in the case of proline and lysine).

CYSTEINE (Fig. 6-1)

Taurine Pathway

Cysteine, after being oxidized by cysteine oxygenase (see Fig. 4-7) to cysteine sulfinate, is decarboxylated to hypotaurine, which is then oxidized further to taurine. The chief physiological function of taurine appears to be conjugation with bile acids, forming the taurocholate family of compounds. In brain and heart, taurine is deaminated to isethionate, a compound of uncertain function.

The overall rate of synthesis of taurine is elevated in experimental muscular necrosis in the rat and is depressed in pyridoxine deficiency. The cysteine sulfinate decarboxylase activity in the livers of male rats is higher than that in females, and, although it is unaffected by castration of males, it is depressed by administration of estrogen to ovariectomized females. Although the decarboxylase utilizes pyridoxal phosphate as coenzyme, the depressed activity seen in pyridoxine deficiency is not remedied by addition of coenzyme *in vitro,* hence reflects a true lowering of apoenzyme levels. These levels in deficient rats can be raised by *in vivo* administration of the vitamin, an effect which is blocked by puromycin. The level of the enzyme is raised by glucocorticoids, and lowered by thyroxine. Although variations in the protein content of the diet have no effect at low levels, a high-protein diet as well as administration of methionine results in a lower level of enzyme.

It would be pleasant to report that the regulation of production of taurine (one of the two conjugants for bile acids), by way of regulation of the decarboxylase, varied with the rate of bile acid production. Unfortunately, it has been observed that the hypothyroid animal, in which the level of decarboxylase is elevated, has a lower rate of cholate production as well as a lower proportion of cholate conjugated with taurine (as against glycine). Thus far it has not been possible to reconcile these findings.

Synthesis of Glutathione

Glutathione is formed in two steps, each catalyzed by a synthetase, each consuming a molecule of ATP. Erythrocyte glutamylcysteine synthetase is inhibited by glutathione and by nicotinamide nucleotides, most strongly NADH, whereas the same enzyme in liver is inhibited by ADP. The glutathione synthetase of both erythrocyte and liver is inhibited by ADP.

Since most of the examples of inhibition mentioned above occur at reasonably physiological concentrations, they probably have functional significance. The role of ADP or glutathione as feedback inhibitors is obvious enough; the same cannot be said of NADH.

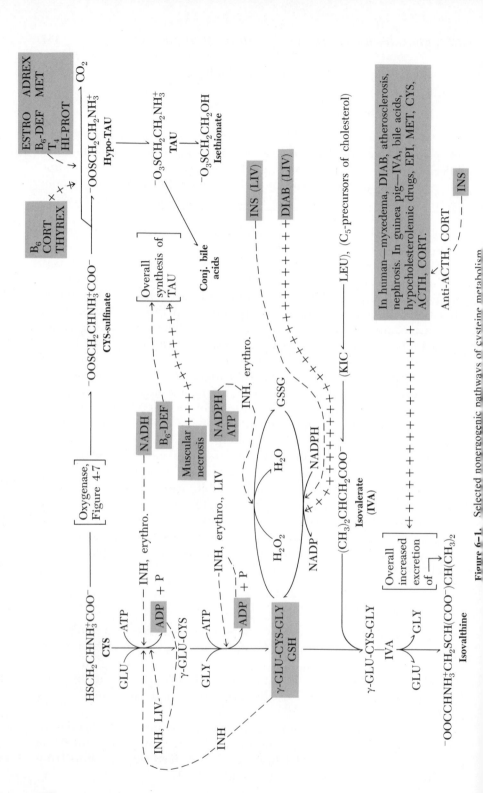

Figure 6–1. Selected nonergogenic pathways of cysteine metabolism.

The reduced form of glutathione is required, for reasons which are not entirely clear, to maintain the integrity of the red blood cell. One protective function is reasonably well established, namely the use of the glutathione peroxidase reaction in the disposal of hydrogen peroxide in the erythrocyte. The oxidized form of glutathione (GSSG) produced in this reaction is reconverted to the reduced form by glutathione reductase, utilizing NADPH as reductant. NADPH is produced in the course of the normal operation of the pentose-shunt pathway of glucose metabolism in the mammalian erythrocyte and not only serves as a cosubstrate in the reduction of GSSG but also has been shown to inhibit red blood cell glutathione peroxidase (as do other nucleotides, such as ATP), thus helping to maintain glutathione in its reduced state. Of course, a contradiction is apparent here, if the peroxidase is regarded as important to the integrity of the red blood cell.

Hepatic glutathione reductase is reduced in level by administration of insulin and elevated in the diabetic. Whether there is any connection between this regulatory mechanism and the presence, in liver, of a glutathione-insulin transhydrogenase which inactivates insulin is not known at this time.

Glutathione as Conjugant: the Isovalthine Pathway*

Although the function of glutathione as a detoxicant of the conjugating variety has been known for many years, e.g., in the synthesis of mercapturic acids, these pathways have been subjected to remarkably little investigation from the viewpoint of regulation. Now that a natural metabolite, isovalerate, has been found to undergo an analogous series of reactions, it is to be hoped that this situation will change for the better.

Isovalerate, arising either as a metabolite of leucine or of the isoprenoid precursors of cholesterol, is conjugated with glutathione in the liver, a thioether bond being formed between the alpha carbon of isovalerate and the cysteinyl moiety of glutathione. Subsequently, and probably in the kidney, the glutamyl and glycyl residues of this intermediate are removed by hydrolysis, forming isovalthine.

Isovalthine is a normal constituent of cat urine, in which its concentration can be greatly increased by administration of leucine to the animal. The compound also is found in the urine of patients treated with the sedative Bromural (alpha-bromoisovalerylurea) and in the urine of patients with a variety of conditions, all having in common the presence of hypercholesterolemia, viz., myxedema (hypothyroidism), diabetes, atherosclerosis, and nephrosis. In guinea pigs, isovalthinuria can be induced by administration of isovalerate, bile acids, hypocholesterolemic drugs, epinephrine, methionine, cysteine, glucocorticoids, and ACTH. Administration of insulin blocks the action of the last two agents mentioned.

---

*For glutathione as possible glutamyl donor in amino acid transport, see footnote on p. 39.

It is evident that most instances of isovalthinuria are caused directly by an increased rate of synthesis of cholesterol, or by blockage of its synthesis, resulting in accumulation of intermediates, or indirectly by agents which increase the rate of mobilization of free fatty acids to the liver (glucocorticoids, epinephrine) with consequent increase in the rate of synthesis of cholesterol.

Whether the rate of production of isovalthine is controlled simply by the rate of supply of raw materials in the foregoing examples or whether there is activation or induction of the conjugating or hydrolytic steps in the synthesis is not known. Also unsettled is the question of the possible contribution of alterations in the rate or extent of catabolism of leucine, e.g., in t1e inborn error of metabolism, isovaleric acidemia, in whic1 at least a part of the excessive accumulation of isovalerate is detoxified by formation of N-isovalerylglycine.

GLYCINE

Purine Pathway (Fig. 6-2)

Figure 6-2 includes only the first few reactions of purine synthesis, sufficient to indicate the involvement of glycine, and the parent nucleo-

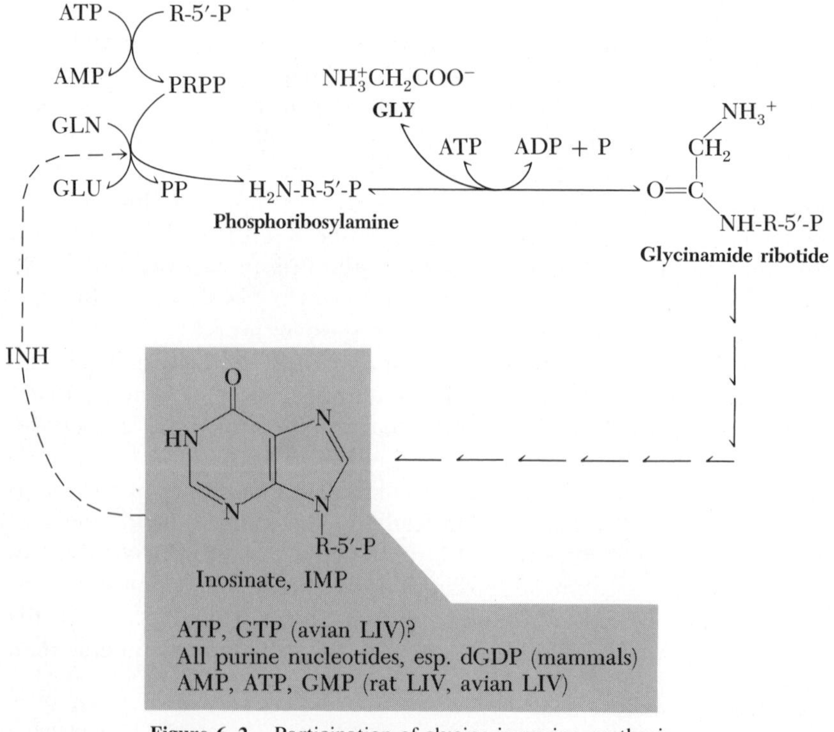

Figure 6–2. Participation of glycine in purine synthesis.

tide of all other purine nucleotides, inosinate. Since they would lead us too far afield from the subject of amino acid metabolism proper, the reactions involved in interconversion of purine nucleotides, catabolism of purines, and synthesis of the various nucleic acids will not be discussed.

Synthesis of purines begins with the formation of phosphoribosyl pyrophosphate, which is then aminated by glutamine under the influence of an amidotransferase, an enzyme subject to feedback regulation in the mammal. The resulting phosphorylated amino sugar condenses with glycine, ATP providing the energy for formation of an amide bond. As can be seen from the structural formulas of glycinamide ribotide and (many reactions later) inosinate, the two carbon atoms and nitrogen of glycine are incorporated contiguously into the purine ring system.

In addition to inosinate, most purine nucleoside mono-, di-, and triphosphates act as metabolite feedback inhibitors of the activity of the amidotransferase in mammalian liver, fibroblasts, various tumors, and in the spleen in virus-induced murine leukemia.

It is of interest that the same site of inhibition is exploited in the chemotherapy of cancer by purine analogs, e.g., 6-mercaptopurine.

Heme Pathway (Fig. 6-3)

The succinyl-CoA-glycine reaction has been discussed briefly previously, as part of the succinate-glycine cycle (see Fig. 4-9). This metabolic scheme, although of dubious ergogenic significance, has been offered as a means of catabolizing glycine, one carbon atom at a time. The involvement of the first reaction of the sequence in the pathway of synthesis of porphyrins and heme undoubtedly is of greater importance to the organism.

The synthesis of porphyrins begins with the condensation of succinyl-CoA and glycine (pyridoxal phosphate being the coenzyme), perhaps forming an unstable intermediate which is immediately decarboxylated to yield delta-aminolevulinate. Following the aminolevulinate synth(et)ase reaction, two molecules of the product condense, under the influence of aminolevulinate dehydratase, to form the monopyrrole, porphobilinogen. As can be seen in the figure, the carboxyl carbon atom of glycine is lost early in the sequence, but the remaining carbon and nitrogen atoms are incorporated into each monopyrrole unit in sets of two.

Additional reactions, which will not be detailed here, lead to the formation of the biologically unimportant series I porphyrinogens and porphyrins, and to the highly significant series III porphyrinogens, protoporphyrin 9, and heme. Combination of four hemes and four globin chains (normally two pairs, e.g., 2 alpha and 2 beta) produces hemoglobin, the major hemoprotein, in terms of amount, in the animal body.

Although aminolevulinate dehydratase is reported to be inhibited by heme, most of the regulatory effects in the porphyrin pathway appear to be directed at the synthase, an enzyme with a short half-life (about 1

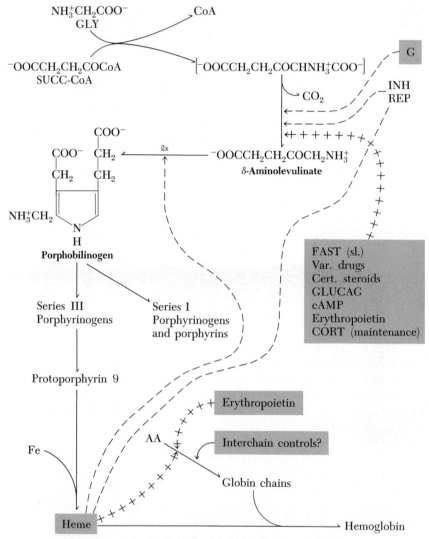

Figure 6–3. Participation of glycine in heme synthesis.

hour in rat mitochondria) and exquisite sensitivity to regulatory influences. The ease with which the normally rate-limiting synthase is induced, such as the ready exacerbation of the tendency toward overproduction of porphyrins in certain types of porphyria (inborn errors of porphyrin metabolism) by ingestion of alcohol or many types of drugs, such as barbiturates, and the ease of production of experimental porphyrias in animals by treatment with a number of chemicals, such as allylisopropylacetamide or dicarbethoxydihydrocollidine, all bespeak the probability that the synthesis of the synthase normally is regulated by a negative (repressor) type of control which is rather sensitive to inactivation or derepression.

Induction of porphyrias in animals by administration of compounds such as allylisopropylacetamide is blocked by administration of NAD, and appears to require the permissive action of glucocorticoids and thyroid hormones.

Returning to more physiological influences, the synthase is induced slightly by fasting and is repressed by a high-glucose diet, effects which are rather unexpected, given the remote connection between heme or hemoglobin synthesis and the major ergogenic pathways.

Although first reported in a nonmammalian system (chick embryo), induction of the synthase by 5β-H steroids such as pregnanolone has since been demonstrated also in the mouse. On the other hand, induction by glucagon in the chick embryo is stated specifically *not* to involve cAMP as intermediary, whereas the synthase is induced readily in rabbit bone marrow cell cultures by very low concentrations of cAMP.

The level of aminolevulinate synthase in isolated perfused rat liver ordinarily decreases rapidly but may be maintained at normal levels through addition of glucocorticoids.

Regulation of the synthase, or of any single enzyme, for that matter, by the hormone erythropoietin is a very complex matter to discuss, since the actions of the hormone also are directed toward the differentiation of erythroid tissue, and it is difficult to disentangle one effect from another. The hormone induces the synthase in mouse spleen and in cultures of bone marrow cells; it may have independent effects on the synthesis of globin chains, as will be discussed shortly.

Negative influences upon the synthase include glucose repression, already mentioned, as well as metabolite repression and inhibition by heme. Objections have been raised on this last point on the basis that inhibition of the synthase in animal cells seems to require concentrations of heme unlikely to be achieved in the cell under normal conditions. However, the synthase functions within the mitochondria, and the last step in heme synthesis, in which iron is attached to protoporphyrin 9 (ferrochelatase reaction), also is intramitochondrial; hence the local, intramitochondrial concentration of heme may well reach that required (approximately 10^{-4} M).

As for developmental regulation of porphyrin synthesis, this pathway of metabolism arises very early in embryonic life, which is to be expected. It is of interest that experimental porphyrias cannot be induced in the fetal rat or mouse.

Although no extensive coverage of the synthesis of globin chains will be attempted, it may be of value to sketch in enough of the subject to indicate the interrelations between the synthesis of heme and that of globin.

In some as yet unexplained manner, four intramitochondrial molecules of newly synthesized heme and four molecules of globin chains (usually two of the alpha and two of the beta type), newly synthesized on cytosolic ribosomes after the usual fashion of proteins, aggregate to form a molecule of hemoglobin. Since it is certain that this agglomeration is not the result of an eight-body collision, regulatory mechanisms must exist to ensure the virtually simultaneous appearance of all eight moieties of the macromolecule at the point of assembly.

In rabbit bone marrow cells and in rabbit reticulocytes there is some evidence for the existence of a pool of alpha chains and a pool of alpha-beta dimers as intermediates in hemoglobin synthesis.

Erythropoietin induces, in bone marrow cells, increased synthesis of RNA, and later, hemoglobin, both preceding the induced increase in cell number. Initially it was believed that the induced RNA was messenger only (for alpha and beta chains), but more recent work has demonstrated induction of many types of RNA under these experimental conditions.

Heme also induces the synthesis of hemoglobin, apparently at the translational level, and possibly by more than one mechanism. On the one hand, heme is reported to stabilize polyribosomes in the rabbit reticulocyte. On the other, there is evidence for the existence of one or more natural inhibitors of globin chain initiation, the formation or activation of which is blocked by heme. In rabbit bone marrow cells and reticulocytes heme promotes the conversion of alpha-beta dimers to hemoglobin tetramers.

Some years ago the suggestion was made that the rate of release of alpha chains from the ribosome is controlled by the availability of beta chains, thus accounting for the equal numbers of these partners-to-be at the site of assembly. However, all recent evidence points to independent synthesis and release of the two types of chains. Nevertheless, some sort of overall regulation exists. It has been shown that, at any given moment in the rabbit reticulocyte, there is 1.5 times more mRNA for alpha than for beta chains associated with ribosomes, but that this factor is balanced by the fact that chain initiation (translation) of the alpha messenger occurs only 65 per cent as often as the beta. It has been suggested that heme functions as a coordinating agent for the synthesis and assembly of alpha and beta chains.

Developmental regulation of hemoglobin synthesis (stressing the globin chains in the molecule) is bound up with regulation of the differentiation of erythroid tissue, meaning, for practical purposes, that virtually nothing is known of the responsible mechanisms. A succession of hemoglobins is seen in the developing mammal, each produced predominantly by a different type of cell. In succession, these are the cells of the yolk sac, liver, and bone marrow. Alpha chains are produced throughout development; the different globins are the result of different partners formed for the alpha chains at each stage. The switching mechanisms for this program are unknown.

The relatively slow adaptation of the mammalian organism to conditions calling for increased synthesis of hemoglobin and increased numbers of erythrocytes (anemia, hypoxia) probably is channeled through erythropoietin. More rapid adaptations must occur through the other inductive and repressive influences operating upon aminolevulinate synthase, in addition to direct negative feedback inhibition by heme. The facilitation of globin synthesis by heme assures the latter that sufficient apoprotein will be formed to provide sites for ligation of prosthetic groups. No reciprocal effect is known; that is, globin chains have not been reported to exert any beneficial effect on the synthesis of heme. The biological rationale of other reported influences on this metabolic pathway, viz., 5β-H steroids, glucocorticoids, glucagon, and cAMP, remains conjectural at this time.

GLUTAMATE (Fig. 6-4)

Glutamine Pathway in Brain and Retina

The synthesis of glutamine in nervous tissue proceeds in the usual manner of other tissues, consuming one pyrophosphate bond of ATP per molecule of amide formed. Glutamate apparently is compartmentalized in brain; that which is directed toward synthesis of glutamine arises from a pool which differs from the glutamate pool drawn upon for the synthesis of gamma-aminobutyrate.

Glutamine synthetase of fetal rat retina is inducible by thyroid hormones from the eighteenth day of gestation until the ninth day after birth, after which the neonate becomes refractory to this stimulus. Unpublished observations also claim neonatal induction in this system by glucocorticoids.

Pig brain glutamine synthetase is inhibited by a number of nucleoside mono-, di-, and triphosphates, glycine, and alanine, and is activated by histidine, but all these effects require concentrations in the millimolar range and are probably devoid of physiological significance. On the other hand, its inhibition by neuraminate (sialate) derivatives in the micromolar range may well be an example of metabolite inhibition, since glutamine is involved in the synthesis of amino sugars which are components of the glycolipids found in the nervous system. Experimentally, the synthetase is inhibited by methionine sulfoximine.

Developmental regulation of the glutamine synthetase in certain nonmammalian systems, e.g., the retina of the chick embryo, has been the object of many investigations which will not be reviewed here. In the rat cerebrum, the enzyme is at a very low level at birth, rises to the adult level in 15 days, and then remains on a plateau. In the cat, each of five areas of the brain shows a different pattern of development, although

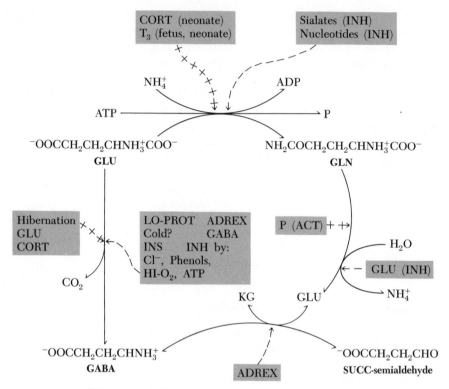

Figure 6–4. Pathways of glutamate in the nervous system.

plateaus of synthetase activity are reached from 6 to 8 weeks after birth in all regions. The enzyme is at a low level in the retina of the fetal rat and does not really begin to develop until the ninth postnatal day, after which it rises 25-fold by the seventeenth day, then remains constant. A close relationship in time has been observed in this system between development of the synthetase and morphological development of the visual structures. Influences of thyroid and glucocorticoid hormones in the rat retina have been noted already.

Reconversion of glutamine to glutamate in the nervous system is catalyzed by a glutaminase which resembles an isoenzyme in kidney in its activation by phosphate and inhibition by glutamate. Although the latter effect may be physiological, as it probably is in kidney, the concentrations of phosphate required for significant activation are about two orders of magnitude greater than the average concentration of this ion in nervous tissue.

Since glutamate has central excitatory properties, whereas glutamine is inert in this regard, it is possible that at least one mechanism for control of the state of excitation of the brain may lie in the balance between the rate of detoxication of glutamate as glutamine and its rate of re-formation through glutaminase. What makes such a proposal doubtful is the plentiful supply of glutamate in the free amino acid pool of nervous tissue and the lack of evidence that its concentration undergoes appreciable fluctuations under physiological conditions. That something of this sort *can* happen, however, is shown by the production of convulsions in animals by administration of methionine sulfoximine, a glutamine synthetase inhibitor which arises from treatment of wheat flour with nitrogen trichloride (a process no longer legal).

Whether glutamine synthetase should be regarded primarily as a pathway of disposal of glutamate, or of ammonia, is of course a moot point. The probable role of brain ammonia in the production of hepatic coma has been discussed previously (Chapter 5).

Gamma-Aminobutyrate Pathway in Brain

Glutamate is decarboxylated in brain by a pyridoxal phosphate–requiring enzyme, forming gamma-aminobutyrate. This product can undergo transamination with ketoglutarate to form succinate semialdehyde, a reaction catalyzed by another enzyme which requires pyridoxal phosphate as coenzyme.

Since the semialdehyde is readily oxidized to succinate, and since glutamate and ketoglutarate are easily interconvertible, it is evident that there exists a possible bypass around the ketoglutarate oxidase system of the Krebs cycle. It is questionable what advantage there could be in such a circumambulation, especially in view of the probable loss in energy which would be sustained. In any event, there is currently no consensus as to the quantitative significance of this pathway.

As mentioned in the previous section, aminobutyrate is formed from glutamate which originates in a metabolic pool different from that which provides the glutamate for synthesis of glutamine. The decarboxylase is elevated during hibernation in rodents and can be induced by administration of fairly large doses of glutamate to mice. Although not inducible to supranormal levels by glucocorticoids, the decreased levels of this enzyme in brain after adrenalectomy can be brought up to normal by administration of the hormones.

The level of the decarboxylase in brain is lowered by adrenalectomy, a low-protein diet, and possibly by exposure to cold or treatment with insulin, these last two effects presumed from the observed diminution in tissue aminobutyrate concentration. There is indirect evidence for repression of synthesis of the decarboxylase by the product, aminobutyrate. The activity of the decarboxylase in rat brain is inhibited by ATP, and the effect is blocked by inorganic phosphate, both at physiological concentrations. The enzyme is inhibited by chloride, also in the physiological range, and by hyperbaric oxygen. Inhibition by certain

phenolic compounds—estrogens, salicylates, phenolic acids of the phen-
ylalanine-tyrosine family—may have no physiological significance, although the last-named group could be involved in the neuropathy of
phenylketonuria.

Despite the nature of its coenzyme, and the fact that the latter is
relatively loosely bound, glutamate decarboxylase is sensitive to few carbonyl-trapping agents *in vivo,* one of the more effective being thiosemicarbazide. Since aminobutyrate exerts central inhibitory effects, convulsions are produced by treatment with semicarbazide, or by deficiency of
pyridoxine, achieved either through direct dietary means or by administration of pyridoxine antimetabolites (e.g., deoxypyridoxine). The con-
vulsive state, in most instances, seems to be related to a diminution in the
concentration of aminobutyrate in the brain.

Glutamate decarboxylase of rat brain exhibits only a low level of activity at birth. A major spurt in development begins about the sixth postnatal day and continues to the eighteenth day, at which point a leveling-
off occurs, followed by a second spurt from day 21 to day 23, at which
adult levels are achieved.

Little can be said concerning the physiological regulation of aminobutyrate transaminase other than it decreases in level following adrenalectomy, along with the decarboxylase. Pyridoxal phosphate is much
more tightly bound to the transaminase than to the decarboxylase,
resulting in immunity of the former to the dietary and chemical treatments which deplete the latter *in vivo.* On the other hand, the transaminase is sensitive to certain carbonyl-trapping agents, such as hydroxylamines and hydrazines, and to the transaminase-inhibitors, cycloserine
and amino-oxyacetate, all of which are effective *in vivo.* Since treatment
with these agents tends to cause accumulation of aminobutyrate, a state
of sedation results.

Development of aminobutyrate transaminase in rat brain appears to
parallel that of the decarboxylase, but with a delay of 3 to 4 days. Succinate semialdehyde dehydrogenase (not shown in Fig. 6-4), on the other
hand, already has almost 30 per cent of the adult activity at the time of
birth of the rat and pursues a somewhat irregular but generally upward
course to reach adult levels at about the same time as the two preceding
enzymes (3 to 4 weeks after birth).

Although it is quite probable that the physiological state of the central nervous system at any given time must be determined by, among
other factors, the instantaneous concentration of aminobutyrate, it is not
entirely clear how the various regulatory influences on the decarboxylase and transaminase contribute to this end. Induction of the decarboxylase by its substrate and repression by its product, and elevation in
level of the decarboxylase during hibernation seem appropriate. On the
other hand, the biological utility of the effects of the glucocorticoids,
protein content of the diet, ATP, inorganic phosphate, oxygen, chloride,
cold, or insulin is not immediately apparent.

ASPARTATE (Fig. 6-5)

N-Acetylaspartate Pathway

Acetylaspartate is found in brain tissue of most vertebrates in high concentration but only in traces in other tissues. Nothing is known of its physiological function, and little is known about its regulation. The observations that urinary excretion of acetylaspartate is greatly increased in the diabetic animal (depancreatized dog, alloxanized rat) and that the compound accumulates in brain homogenates inhibited by fluoroacetate have led to the conclusion that synthesis of acetylaspartate is increased in conditions characterized by excessive formation or accumulation of acetyl-CoA. Since acetylaspartate does not pass the blood-brain barrier, but rather is synthesized *in situ*, it seems probable that the foregoing observations are the result of events transpiring within the brain, where aspartate perhaps acts as an "acetyl sink," taking up the surplus which occurs in certain conditions.

Asparagine Pathway

In most mammalian systems which have been investigated, asparagine is synthesized by the reaction of aspartate with glutamine (which generally has been found superior to free ammonia as cosubstrate), the energy for the amidation being supplied by the cleavage of ATP to AMP and pyrophosphate.

The level of asparagine synthetase is elevated in rat liver during regeneration, in tumor-bearing animals, and in conditions leading to generally low levels of asparagine in the organism, such as dietary restriction of the amide or treatment by injection of asparaginase. *In vitro* investigations have shown that the synthetase from normal tissues and from some tumors is susceptible to product inhibition by asparagine, although the enzyme from guinea pig liver is said to be resistant. Evidence for product *repression* also has been obtained.

The major pathway for reconversion of asparagine to aspartate appears to be simple hydrolysis, catalyzed by asparaginase. Great interest is now centered on this enzyme, since its injection has a therapeutic effect on some leukemias and lymphoid tumors. Its mechanism of action apparently depends upon a nutritional requirement for the amide on the part of certain tumors, caused by either complete absence of the synthetase or its presence at a low level, not inducible (or derepressible) to higher levels by lack of asparagine.

The level of asparaginase is reduced in regenerating liver, a system in which reciprocal effects are shown by the synthetase and hydrolase. Unfortunately, the influences of hormones and diet on asparaginase seem to vary with the species under investigation. Thus, estrogens

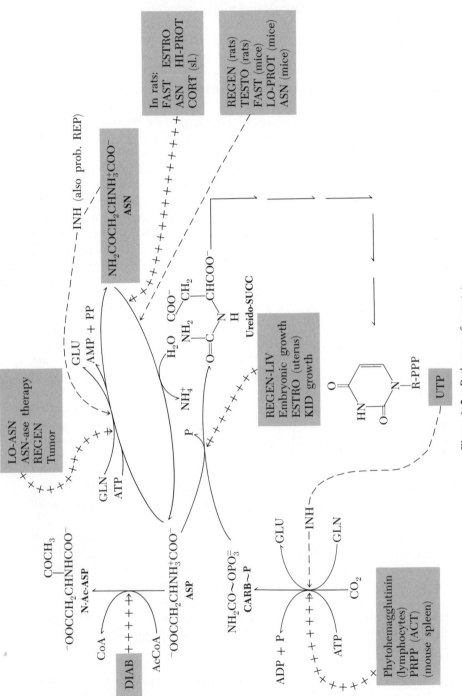

Figure 6–5. Pathways of aspartate.

increase and androgens decrease the level of asparaginase in the livers of rats, explaining observed sex differences; in mice, no sex differences are seen in this enzyme. Although adrenalectomy has no effect, administration of glucocorticoids to rats has a small inducing effect on the hepatic asparaginase. Starvation causes an increase in the enzyme level in rat liver, after an initial slight decrease, whereas the enzyme in mouse liver progressively decreases. A low-protein diet has no effect in the rat but causes a small decrease in the mouse. A high-protein diet induces the enzyme in rats, but no change is seen in mice. Injection of asparagine slowly induces the enzyme in rats, whereas aspartate has no effect. Both compounds depress the level of the enzyme slightly in mice.

Observations in man and other mammals indicate great constancy in the concentration of asparagine in the plasma, suggesting the operation of homeostatic mechanisms. In the rat, the level of this compound in plasma is maintained by hepatic synthesis and addition to the plasma when the level falls, and by hepatic hydrolysis and oxidation of aspartate, after deamination, via the Krebs cycle, when the plasma level rises above the norm.

The rat embryo has a fairly high asparagine synthetase activity, but no asparaginase. Postnatal development is characterized by decrease of the former and increase of the latter. In rat liver, asparaginase appears immediately after birth, increases for 5 days, remains on a level for about a week, then increases again to reach nearly adult levels at 20 days. The early increase is induced by intake of food, since starvation caused by separation from the mother blocks it. The second developmental spurt is enhanced by glucocorticoids (adrenocortical function increases after the tenth postnatal day in the rat). Attempts at prenatal evocation of asparaginase by injection of glucocorticoids, glucagon, asparagine, or an amino acid mixture into the fetus have been unsuccessful.

It is quite probable that asparagine is an essential amino acid for most animal cells, with the exception of those supplied with the synthetase, such as liver and certain tumors. It follows that liver probably is the source of this compound for the other tissues of the body, thus accounting for the constancy of concentration of asparagine in the plasma and the synthetase-hydrolase balance of activities provided by the liver. In the embryonic state and during liver regeneration, when synthesis of new tissue and new protein proceeds at a high rate, the level of synthetase should be high and that of asparaginase should be low or absent. It also seems appropriate that maturation should remove much (but not all) of the requirement for supplies of asparagine to the tissues, whereas the constant influx of the amide in the diet requires that appreciable amounts of asparaginase be present in order to maintain a physiological balance. Unfortunately, little comparable sense can be made of the regulatory effects of hormones or diet, particularly in view of the odd species variations.

Pyrimidine Pathway

In animal cells, the synthesis of pyrimidines begins with the formation of carbamyl phosphate, catalyzed by an extramitochondrial synthetase which utilizes glutamine as the source of ammonia. (This enzyme is quite distinct from that which is involved in the ornithine cycle.) In the second step, the carbamyl group is transferred to aspartate by aspartate transcarbamylase, forming carbamyl aspartate or ureidosuccinate. After a number of intervening reactions, the parent of the pyrimidine nucleotides is produced, uridylate (UMP). It will be noted that aspartate contributes to the pyrimidine ring three carbon atoms and one nitrogen atom, the fourth carbon atom of aspartate being lost in a decarboxylation step. The pyrimidine nucleoside monophosphate is transformed readily to the triphosphate (UTP), which is pictured in Figure 6-5 since it plays an important regulatory role.

In contrast to bacterial cells, mammalian cells regulate the synthesis of pyrimidines primarily through the carbamyl phosphate synthetase reaction. The enzyme is increased in level in the human lymphocyte when blastogenesis is induced by treatment with phytohemagglutinin. In the same cell system, the activity of the enzyme is inhibited by uridine triphosphate, an example of negative feedback found also in the enzyme in fetal and adult rat liver, mouse spleen, ascites cells, and ascites hepatoma. It is interesting to note that N-acetylglutamate, the activator of the intramitochondrial synthetase, is without effect on the enzyme of the pyrimidine pathway. However, the synthetase from hematopoietic mouse spleen is strongly activated by phosphoribosyl pyrophosphate.

Influenced by the findings in bacteria, early investigators of the aspartate transcarbamylase in mammals reported instances of negative feedback inhibition by various pyrimidine and even purine nucleotides. Most recent papers flatly contradict the earlier work. In fact, assays of the comparative specific activities of the synthetase and transcarbamylase in mammalian tissues have shown the former to be rate-limiting, and therefore the logical candidate for regulatory influences. Aspartate transcarbamylase is subject to induction in certain circumstances. These examples all fall in the category of conditions of increased mitotic rate; the level of the transcarbamylase is elevated in the embryo, in regenerating liver, in compensatory renal growth following unilateral nephrectomy, and in the uterus (of the immature rat) stimulated to growth by estrogen. Fasting and refeeding have little effect on the enzyme in rat liver.

Both the carbamyl phosphate synthetase and the transcarbamylase are functional in fetal tissues at a developmental stage when the ornithine cycle (initiated by a different carbamyl phosphate synthetase) is absent. In rat liver, the transcarbamylase decreases from the high level which it attains in the late fetal stage, to gradually lower levels after birth, and eventually to the final quite low levels characteristic of the adult. In rat heart the enzyme suddenly drops to one-half its previous value at birth, then later decreases to practically zero activity in the adult.

Since the pyrimidine pathway properly belongs to the area of nucleic acid metabolism, one might expect to encounter regulatory mechanisms appropriate to attune the rate of synthesis of pyrimidines to the demands of cell growth and replication. The cited induction of the synthetase in lymphocytes stimulated to differentiate, as well as the instances of elevation of the transcarbamylase paralleling the mitotic rate, is in accord with these expectations. Inhibition of the synthetase by UTP, finally, insures that the rate of production of pyrimidine nucleotides does not exceed their rate of utilization.

ARGININE: CREATINE PATHWAY (Fig. 6-6)

The synthesis of creatine consists of two steps: first, a reversible transfer of the amidine group of arginine to glycine, and second, an irreversible transmethylation of the resulting guanidoacetate (also called glycocyamine) to yield creatine.

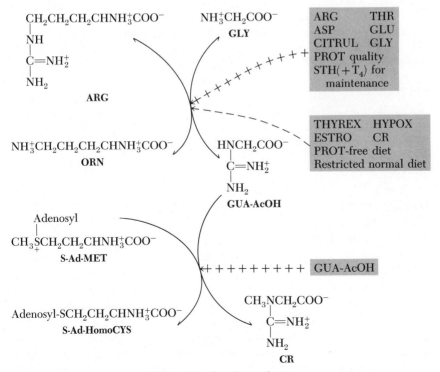

Figure 6–6. Creatine pathway.

Early investigations on creatine synthesis were confined to the rat and certain other laboratory animals in which transamidinase activity was absent from the liver. This finding gave rise to the generalization that two tissues were required for the complete synthesis of creatine, one (such as kidney) for the transamidinase step, and another (chiefly the liver) for the transmethylation. Actually, even in the rat, both enzymes are found together in many tissues, such as kidney, pancreas, brain, and testis. In the rat, the transamidinase is found additionally in the spleen, skeletal muscle, and heart muscle. Although rat liver contains transmethylase, as mentioned, transamidinase activity is absent. In the human, both enzymes are present in liver, kidney, brain, pancreas, and spleen.

The involvement of creatine in the storage of energy as phosphocreatine, and the transformation of both the former and latter to creatinine, are outside the purview of this discussion. However, it should be noted that one site important in both transformations is skeletal muscle, in which (since there is no *in situ* synthesis of creatine due to absence of the transmethylase) transport mechanisms for creatine may well be the controlling factors in its metabolism, as discussed in Chapter 3.

In the kidney of the weaning rat, the level of transamidinase is elevated by supplementation of the diet with arginine, threonine, or aspartate. The decreases in level of the enzyme caused by creatine supplementation, protein-free diet, or restricted intake of normal diet (all discussed below) are counteracted by, respectively, glycine, arginine, threonine, or citrulline in the first instance, and arginine or glycine in the second and third. It has also been observed that the level of rat kidney transamidinase reflects the nutritional quality of the dietary protein.

Kidneys of male rats contain a higher concentration of transamidinase than those of females, an effect due more to the absence of a repressive influence of estrogens in the male than to an apparently feeble positive effect of androgens. Growth hormone is required for maintenance of the normal level of transamidinase but is effective only in the presence of thyroid hormone.

In the area of negative influences on the transamidinase, it may be mentioned that much work has been done in nonmammalian systems, such as the liver of the chick or chick embryo. The repressive influence of creatine in these systems, which has been known for some years, recently has been characterized as unphysiological, requiring pharmacological doses of creatine. It also has been reported that, in the early chick embryo, the level of the enzyme rises in parallel with the level of creatine. As for mammalian systems, dietary supplementation with creatine represses the transamidinase in rat, rabbit, and mouse kidney, rat pancreas, and decidual tissue of the pregnant rat. The repressive effect of vitamin E deficiency in the rabbit is ascribed to the excessive amounts of creatine presented to the kidney for excretion in this condition. Other negative dietary influences already mentioned are the protein-free diet and restricted intake of a normal diet, the effects of which, as well as the effects of creatine supplementation, are reversible by administration of specific amino acids.

Endocrine regulatory factors include the repressive influence of estrogens noted previously as well as the negative effects resulting from removal of those endocrine tissues responsible for normally positive effects—thyroidectomy and hypophysectomy.

Where studied, it has been found that the alterations in transamidinase level are rather slow. In accord with this, the half-life of rat kidney transamidinase has been determined to be 38 hours.

Although the transmethylase enzyme, when it has been assayed along with the transamidinase after any of the previously mentioned experimental procedures, has shown no change, it has been reported recently to be induced in rat liver after dietary supplementation with one of its substrates, guanidoacetate. Additional recent data suggest that the specific activity of the transmethylase may be considerably less than that of the transamidinase. If so, then the transmethylase may be rate-limiting, and future investigations of regulation might profitably be directed toward this enzyme rather than the other.

Despite considerable interest in the synthesis of creatine in the embryo, especially in nonmammalian forms, there has been little systematic study of developmental aspects of the two participating enzymes. It has been shown that, late in gestation, the transmethylase activity of the fetal rat liver is less than half that of the maternal organ.

Insofar as the rationale of regulation of the creatine pathway is concerned, metabolite repression of the transamidinase and substrate induction of the transmethylase do not stand out as unusual. Those amino acids which counteract the repressive effect of creatine may be doing so via a disguised inductive effect of their own, not ordinarily demonstrable, with arginine and glycine acting as substrate inducers, citrulline and threonine acting as sources of these two substrates, respectively. The action of aspartate is not readily explained. The dietary effects of quality and quantity of protein perhaps are related to the need for more creatine in protein-anabolic states, in which the major mass of new protein is laid down in skeletal muscle. In harmony with this hypothesis are the positive effect of growth hormone and the negative effect of thyroid. Although one might expect a positive effect also from androgen, for some unknown reason this system operates primarily through negative effects of estrogen.

HISTIDINE: HISTAMINE PATHWAY (Fig. 6-7)

Histidine is converted to histamine by a simple decarboxylation; the coenzyme of the decarboxylase is pyridoxal phosphate. The resulting amine may follow either of two pathways. In one, the amine is oxidized

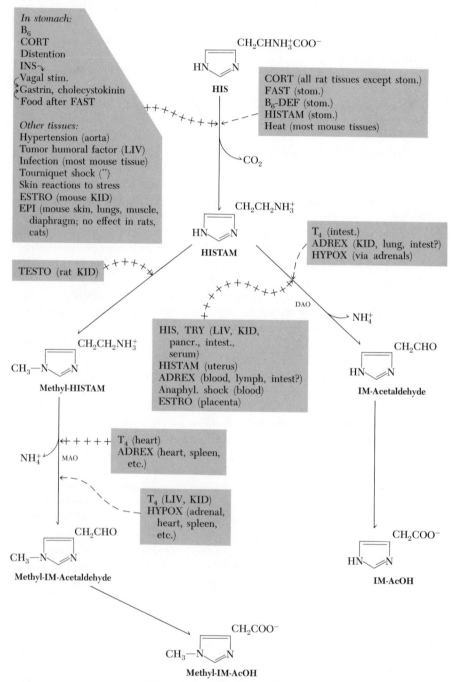

Figure 6–7. Histamine pathway.

to the corresponding aldehyde by histaminase (diamine oxidase), the aldehyde is oxidized to a carboxylic acid by an aldehyde dehydrogenase, and the resulting imidazoleacetate excreted as such, as the ribotide, or as the riboside. In the alternate pathway, histamine is first methylated, then oxidized in two steps to the product, methylimidazoleacetate, the first step being catalyzed by monoamine oxidase, the second by an aldehyde dehydrogenase as in the first pathway.

Study of the regulation of the decarboxylation of histidine to histamine is complicated by the existence, in many tissues, of a relatively nonspecific aromatic amino acid decarboxylase which attacks histidine, although it is much more effective with substrates such as dihydroxyphenylalanine (DOPA) or 5-hydroxytryptophan. A truly specific histidine decarboxylase is found in fetal tissues, placenta, gastric mucosa, red bone marrow, and in certain tumors. Mast cells are particularly rich in this enzyme, as are certain enterochromaffin-like cells in the stomach. Fortunately, the specific decarboxylase differs from the nonspecific in a number of properties: its pH optimum is lower, its K_m for histidine is lower, and its action is not potentiated by benzene. These characteristics usually have enabled investigators to state that a given regulatory influence is exerted upon the specific decarboxylase when both enzymes are found together in a tissue.

The level of histidine decarboxylase in gastric mucosa is elevated by administration of pyridoxine derivatives, which, in addition to providing the coenzyme, have a true inducing action on the apoenzyme *in vivo*. Induction also follows administration of glucocorticoids, and various stimuli which either directly excite secretory mechanisms of the stomach (gastrin, cholecystokinin) or operate via parasympathetic stimulation, viz., distention of stomach wall, administration of parasympathomimetic compounds (carbachol), vagal stimulation, insulin (functioning via hypoglycemic vagal stimulation), and refeeding fasted animals.

A humoral factor produced by tumors induces the decarboxylase in liver, whereas hypertension does the same for the enzyme of the aorta. The skin of the mouse and rat reacts to stresses with a local increase in level of histidine decarboxylase. Estrogens are reported to induce it in the mouse kidney. More general are the effects of infection or tourniquet shock, which raise the level of the enzyme in most tissues of the mouse. The influence of catecholamines appears to be species-specific; these hormones are inducers of the decarboxylase in the skin, lungs, muscle, and diaphragm of the mouse but have no such effects in the rat or cat.

In contrast to their action on rat stomach, glucocorticoid hormones are repressors of the decarboxylase in all other tissues. As could be anticipated from the foregoing discussion, the level of the enzyme in the gastric mucosa falls during fasting or pyridoxine deficiency. It also decreases in most tissues of the mouse exposed to excessive environmental heat. Although the evidence has been slow in accumulating, it now appears that histamine, the product of the reaction, acts as repressor of the decarboxylase in the gastric mucosa.

Diamine oxidase (histaminase), the initial enzyme in one of the two pathways of disposal of histamine shown in Figure 6-7, is induced in liver, pancreas, kidney, and intestine (and rises in serum) after administration of histidine or tryptophan. Histamine itself induces the enzyme in the uterus, as do estrogens in the placenta. Levels of the oxidase in blood are increased by adrenalectomy and by anaphylactic shock. The effect of adrenalectomy on the level of enzyme in the intestine is the subject of directly contradictory reports.

Diamine oxidase of intestine is repressed by thyroid hormones. Adrenalectomy reduces the level of the enzyme in kidney and lung; the disagreement with respect to intestine has been mentioned. Hypophysectomy results in a lower level of oxidase in the intestine and kidney.

The initial enzyme of the alternate pathway, imidazole-N-methyltransferase, is induced in rat kidney by androgens.

Monoamine oxidase, which probably is of even greater importance in the catabolism of indoleamines and catecholamines, will be discussed only briefly at this point. It is induced in heart by thyroid hormones and is increased in level in heart, spleen, and other tissues by adrenalectomy. It is decreased in level in liver and kidney by thyroid hormones, and in adrenal, heart, spleen, and other tissues by hypophysectomy.

Histidine decarboxylase levels are low in the liver and kidney of the fetal guinea pig but rise shortly before birth to adult values. Of the common laboratory animals, only the rat and guinea pig have significant hepatic decarboxylase activity in the late fetal stage; this is not found in the mouse, hamster, or rabbit. The enzyme remains low postnatally in the rat after peaking on the seventeenth day of gestation, but levels increase in the other species. The fetal rat liver enzyme resembles in properties the bone marrow decarboxylase of the adult rat and follows a pattern in development parallel with that of hepatosplenal hematopoiesis. It is suggested that histamine may have something to do with the latter process. In the human infant, decarboxylase activity is low in the liver and kidney in the fetal stage, but it increases sharply at term.

The levels of diamine oxidase in various tissues are reported to increase with age. In pregnant women, the enzyme level is low in the amniotic fluid in the first weeks of gestation, increases markedly about the twentieth week, reaches a peak in the thirty-fourth week, and then decreases sharply toward term. No similar pattern is seen in the fetus.

Little is known of the development of the imidazole-N-methyltransferase. It is absent from the 19- to 24-week-old human fetus.

Monoamine oxidase increases in the heart with age. In the guinea pig, which is well developed functionally at birth, the brain monoamine oxidase concentration is almost at an adult level in the newborn. On the other hand, in the rat, which is relatively much less mature at birth, brain monoamine oxidase is at a low level in the neonate, develops slowly for the first 10 days, then increases more rapidly to reach adult levels several weeks after birth.

COLLAGEN PATHWAY OF PROLINE AND LYSINE (Fig. 6-8)

Synthesis of collagen is a function of the fibroblast, the cell in which the polypeptide chains which will ultimately form the final protein are assembled on polyribosomes in the usual manner. However, there are several unusual features in this process, one being the peculiar composition of the final protein. Collagen is characterized by a high content of glycine and proline, and by having in its composition two amino acids, hydroxyproline and hydroxylysine, for which there exist no transfer RNA's. These hydroxylated amino acids are not incorporated into the peptide chains at the stage of translation; the chains as produced contain unhydroxylated proline and lysine. At this stage the protein is known as *protocollagen.*

Hydroxylation of protocollagen is believed to be the rate-limiting step in collagen synthesis. Certain prolyl and lysyl residues are attacked by specific hydroxylases utilizing molecular oxygen, requiring ascorbate and ferrous iron as cofactors and coupled with the oxidation of ketoglutarate to succinate. Once hydroxylated, three peptide chains combine to form a monomeric molecule, in which are found two peptide chains with identical amino acid composition (alpha$_1$) and a third with somewhat different composition (alpha$_2$), each chain twisted into a left-handed helix, with the cable of all three chains twisted into a right-handed superhelix. At this stage, each peptide chain is longer than those eventually extruded from the cell, the extensions being at the N-terminals. Since there is some evidence for the presence of cystine (which is absent from interstitial collagen) in these extensions, it is possible that formation of the triple helix is facilitated initially by disulfide bonds.

At some point during its existence, but before extrusion from the cell, the collagen precursor is glycosylated. Galactosyl and glucosyl residues are transferred from their linkages with uridine diphosphate to hydroxyl groups on hydroxylysine. The now hydroxylated, glycosylated but still extension-bearing precursor molecule which is ready for export has been called *procollagen* or *transport form.*

Extrusion from the cell, by as yet undetermined mechanisms, exposes the procollagen to enzymatic cleavage of the extensions. The smaller collagen precursor thus produced is *tropocollagen.* Electrostatic interactions among groups in the side chains of amino acid residues in the now-exposed N-terminal regions of adjacent molecules lead to aggregation into fibrils.

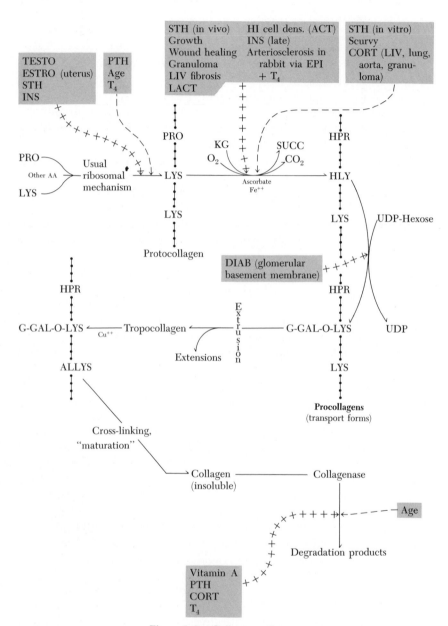

Figure 6–8. Collagen pathway.

Macroscopic fibers formed of aggregated tropocollagen molecules which have undergone no chemical alterations beyond those just described have little tensile strength and resemble the abnormal collagens found in certain pathological conditions. Formation of true connective tissue collagen requires one further modification, aging or maturation, a process involving cross-linking.

A few lysyl residues are oxidatively deaminated (on the free epsilon amino group) by lysyl oxidase, which probably requires cupric ion as cofactor. The resultant aldehyde derivative of lysine, sometimes called allysine, participates in the formation of aldol and Schiff base cross-links, which are characteristic of the gradually more insoluble and more mature collagen fibrils. Some of these cross-links are intramolecular; coupling of two alpha chains produces a beta chain of twice the original weight. Other cross-links are intermolecular and help to convert the protein to a complex, three-dimensional network required for its role as the backbone of various types of connective tissue.

Little is known of the enzymatic catabolism of collagen. Native (undenatured) collagen is resistant to digestion by trypsin but is susceptible to the hydrolytic action of certain lysosomal cathepsins functioning at acid pH's, an apparently nonlysosomal collagenase with an acid pH optimum produced by skin fibroblasts and a collagenase with a neutral pH optimum made by bone explants in culture. This last enzyme is produced in the form of a latent procollagenase, activated by a protease.

Although it is difficult to differentiate the influence of certain factors at the sites of transcription and translation from their influence on the hydroxylation and later stages of collagen synthesis, there is some evidence that peptide synthesis as such (i.e., formation of protocollagen) is induced by androgens, growth hormone, and insulin (and estrogen in the uterus), and is repressed by age, parathyroid hormone, and thyroid hormones.

The rate-limiting hydroxylation of protocollagen (as measured by formation of hydroxyproline in the protein) is promoted by *in vivo* administration of growth hormone, although it has been concluded that this effect must be indirect, since the hormone exerts a negative effect upon hydroxylation *in vitro* in various fractions of collagen in guinea pig granuloma and in skin and bone of the weanling rat; in these systems unhydroxylated protocollagen continues to be synthesized. On the other hand, it is well established that the level of protocollagen proline hydroxylase is elevated in conditions of growth or tissue repair, such as in growing fetal tissue, wound healing, experimental granuloma, and experimental liver fibrosis. The enzyme also is increased in cultures of fibroblasts when these reach a condition of high cell density; the phenomenon is one of activation, not induction, in this case. Of considerable medical interest is the observation that the hydroxylase is elevated in the aorta of rabbits in which hypertension has been induced by administration of epinephrine and thyroxine, the rise in enzyme activity accompanying the development of atheromatous plaques. Insulin, which has some of the characteristics of a growth hormone, exerts a late positive effect on the hydroxylase in cultures of newborn rat bone, following an early phase in which the hormone stimulates simple incorporation of proline (not hydroxylation) into collagen. Collagen synthesis in cultured fibroblasts is stimulated by lactate, probably at the protocollagen proline hydroxylase step. The enzyme is induced in livers of rats and baboons subjected to long-term administration of ethanol, possibly via the resulting known increase in NADH concentration in the liver and the consequently increased production of lactate. How lactate functions is not known.

The negative *in vitro* influence of growth hormone on the hydroxylation has been mentioned already. Although not truly a regulatory mechanism, it should be noted that, as expected, hydroxylation is impaired in scurvy, since ascorbate is a cofactor of the reaction. The most significant physiological regulators of the hydroxylase reaction are the glucocorticoid hormones, which repress protocollagen proline hydroxylation in liver, lung, and experimental granuloma. The anti-inflammatory effect of glucocorticoids on granuloma correlates with the reduction in hydroxylase levels in the granuloma tissue. These hormones have no effect on the enzyme in fetal liver explants.

Little is known of the regulation of the subsequent steps of collagen synthesis or maturation. The activity of the transglycosylases is elevated in the glomerular basal membrane of the human diabetic, possibly leading to "overglycosylation," which, by interfering with the normal mode of packing of collagen fibers, could account for the thickening of the membrane which is observed in this condition. No regulatory influences have been reported which act directly upon the lysyl oxidase or cross-linking steps (the latter being nonenzymatic).

Our knowledge of the regulation of the catabolism of collagen is not in a very satisfactory state. Thyroid hormone appears to accelerate the breakdown of collagen, although it is not established that its site of action is specifically one of the collagenases. Taken together with its negative influence on the translation step and its positive influence on proline hydroxylation, it seems that thyroid hormone promotes both anabolism and catabolism of collagen, or *turnover*.

The activities of glucocorticoid hormones are more consistent. In addition to repression of the hydroxylation step in various tissues, these hormones induce the appearance of a collagenase with acid pH optimum in fibroblasts from human or mouse skin. Addition of purified collagenase to these cultures blocks the induction, suggestive of a feedback control mechanism.

The role of vitamin A in collagen metabolism is not at all clear. According to some, this vitamin promotes the release of lysosomal "collagenases." It is known that the procollagenase of bone and skin, which becomes a neutral collagenase, can be activated by lysosomes. Whatever its specific site of action may be, the general influence of vitamin A on collagen is in the catabolic direction.

There have been no systematic studies of the development of the collagen-synthesizing enzymes in the mammal. However, collagen, in the form of various types of connective tissue, appears early in embryonic life, hence the requisite enzymes must be present. It has been reported that less mature and more soluble forms of collagen predominate in the young embryo, becoming more fibrillar and less soluble with age. In contrast to the significant rate of synthesis of collagen in embryonic life, this protein has one of the lowest rates of turnover in the adult. As a generalization, it is often stated that collagenase activity decreases with age, probably as one facet of decreased turnover.

As an important structural constituent of the organism, collagen could be expected to be subject to many of the regulatory factors which usually are found to play roles in the general pathways of anabolism and catabolism of protein. In accord with this expectation are the collagen-anabolic influences of growth hormone (discounting the anomalous *in vitro* findings), insulin, androgen, and estrogen in the uterus, as well as the catabolic effects of glucocorticoid and thyroid hormones. The anti-anabolic effect of parathyroid hormone on collagen metabolism complements its action on calcified tissue; by breaking down the collagen framework, osteoclastic activity is facilitated and calcium is released. On the other hand, no rationale can be suggested at this time for the reported effects of epinephrine, vitamin A, or the diabetic state.

METHIONINE

Methyl Group Pathways (Fig. 6-9)

S-Adenosylmethionine, the chief transmethylating agent of the organism, is formed by activation of methionine through addition of the adenosyl moiety of ATP to the sulfur atom of the amino acid, splitting out from the nucleotide pyrophosphate and orthophosphate groups in the process. The sulfonium pole thus produced confers considerable group-transfer potential to the three attached fragments, although it is only the methyl with which we are concerned at this point.

After the activation reaction, methyl transfers can occur to many receptors, both physiological and foreign. The remaining demethylated agent, S-adenosylhomocysteine, loses its adenosyl moiety through hydrolysis, leaving homocysteine. This last compound lacks only a methyl group to become methionine again. The requisite fragment is supplied by either of two pathways: one, a simple transmethylation from betaine,

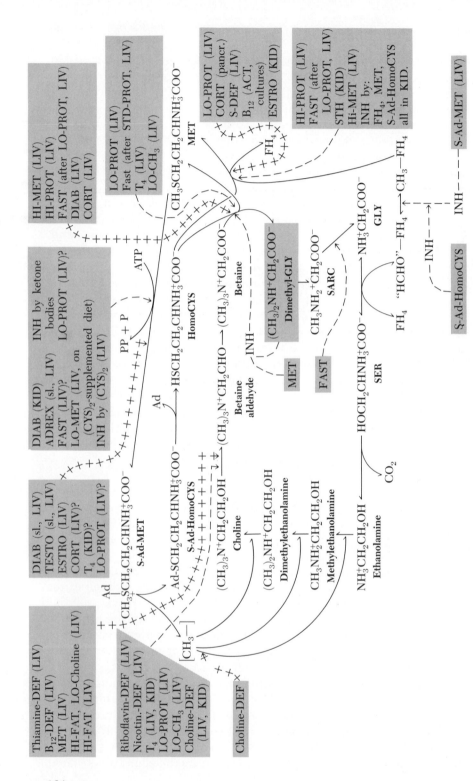

Figure 6–9. Methyl group pathways.

a transmethylating agent derived from the ethanolamine family of compounds; the other, a more complex sequence of reactions involving the *de novo* synthesis of methyl groups from one-carbon fragments on the formate or formaldehyde level of oxidation. Since both of these pathways are joined in a cyclic pattern of reactions interconnecting many compounds of physiological interest and characterized, in part, by interconversions of various forms of one-carbon fragments, they will be presented in some detail.

Beginning the cycle at serine, it may be noted that the decarboxylation of this amino acid to form ethanolamine and the stepwise methylation of the latter (utilizing S-adenosylmethionine as the source of methyl groups) to eventually form choline all occur while the named reactants exist as constituents of phospholipids. Oxidation of free choline, first to betaine aldehyde, then to betaine, provides another onium type of transmethylating agent, which, after donating one of its methyl groups to homocysteine, forms dimethylglycine. Conversion of dimethylglycine to sarcosine (monomethylglycine) and of the latter to glycine requires the successive removal of two methyl groups, but at the oxidation level of formaldehyde. The glycine thus produced, by addition of a formaldehyde (methylene) group (carried as a one-carbon fragment on the coenzyme, tetrahydrofolate), yields serine and thus completes the cycle.

Although not indicated in Figure 6-9, the compound of formaldehyde-tetrahydrofolate is in metabolic equilibrium with analogous tetrahydrofolate compounds bearing one-carbon fragments on the oxidation level of formate. In the reductive direction, which is of greater relevance to the pathways under discussion, formaldehyde-tetrahydrofolate is interconvertible with methyl-tetrahydrofolate. Under the influence of a specific transmethylase, this methyl group is transferred to homocysteine to form methionine. The mechanism of the reaction is complex and not yet entirely clarified, but it is known that the methyl group is carried transiently by a cobamide coenzyme (derived from vitamin B_{12}). S-Adenosylmethionine is required as activator.

In view of the metabolic importance of the methionine-activating reaction, it is surprising how few regulatory mechanisms have been found which are well established and noncontroversial. The level of the enzyme in liver is increased slightly in alloxan diabetes and by androgen, more significantly by estrogen (there is one claim that androgen exerts a negative influence). According to some, glucocorticoids are generally inducers of the enzyme, whereas others find such effects only in the neonatal rat. Renal methionine-activating enzyme is said by one laboratory to be induced by thyroid hormones, although another report claims no effect is produced. Contradictory findings also are seen after low-protein diets (increase or decrease) and after fasting (decrease or no effect) in the case of liver enzyme.

As indicated previously, low-protein diets and fasting *may* have negative effects on the level of the activating enzyme in liver. Alloxan diabetes decreases the level of the enzyme in kidney, and adrenalectomy has a slight influence in the same direction in the case of the liver. The liver enzyme also is repressed on diets which are low in methionine and supplemented with cystine. Cystine itself has an inhibitory effect on the activity of the enzyme, as have ketone bodies.

Since the K_m for methionine is about 1 mM and the concentration of methionine in liver is about 40 to 100 μM, the rate of operation of the activating enzyme in the last analysis may well be controlled by the hepatic level of substrate.

Regulation of certain transmethylations from S-adenosylmethionine will be discussed in connection with metabolic pathways to be taken up later, such as the catecholamines and indoleamines. In the pathway shown in Figure 6-9, methylation of the ethanolamines to yield choline is induced by a choline-deficient diet.

Choline oxidase is an intramitochondrial enzyme which is subject to many regulatory influences. At least a part of its oxidative activity toward choline in liver mitochondria is coupled to oxidative phosphorylation, hence to this extent the enzyme presumably is controlled by the various factors operative in the domain of mitochondrial energy production.

The level of the oxidase in liver is greatly influenced by diet. It is elevated by high-fat or high-fat low-choline diets, and further by methionine (or glycine plus homocysteine) on the latter diet. Similar increases are seen in deficiencies of thiamine or vitamin B_{12}.

In the opposite direction, lower levels of liver oxidase are found on diets deficient in choline (in this case, kidney enzyme also), protein, and methyl donors in general, or in the vitamins nicotinamide or riboflavin. Fairly long adherence to a choline-deficient diet is required in order to lower the level of the oxidase; short-term experiments may have no effect. Thyroid hormones are reported to repress the oxidase in both liver and kidney.

The betaine-homocysteine transmethylation reaction is subject to a number of controls. The enzyme in liver is induced by a methionine load, high-protein diet, fasting after a low-protein diet, alloxan diabetes, and glucocorticoids. It is repressed by fasting after a "standard" diet, low-protein diet, a diet deficient in methyl donors, or by thyroid hormones. The activity of the enzyme is inhibited by the two products, methionine and dimethylglycine.

Little is known of the regulation of most other reactions of the cycle under consideration, other than that the sarcosine dehydrogenase level of rat liver is decreased by fasting.

The reductase which converts the fragment carried by tetrahydrofolate from the formaldehyde to the methyl level of oxidation in liver is inhibited by S-adenosylmethionine; the inhibition is in turn blocked by S-adenosylhomocysteine.

As noted previously, the enzyme catalyzing transfer of a methyl group from methyl-tetrahydrofolate to homocysteine requires a cobamide (vitamin B_{12}) coenzyme and is activated by S-adenosylmethionine. It is also activated in cultures of various types of mammalian cells by the addition of vitamin B_{12}. The hepatic enzyme is present in higher concentration in the liver of the male rat than in the female, although in kidney the transmethylase is induced by estrogen. Low-protein and sulfur-deficient diets increase the level of the enzyme in liver; glucocorticoids do the same in pancreas.

The activity of the renal transmethylase is inhibited by tetrahydrofolate, S-adenosylhomocysteine, and methionine. Repression of the liver enzyme is caused by a high-protein diet, fasting after a low-protein diet, and a methionine load. The kidney enzyme is repressed by growth hormone.

The methionine-activating enzyme of rat liver is present in the late fetal stage at a concentration of 58 to 100 per cent that of the adult but undergoes an even greater increase in the neonate. Although the postnatal rise is said to be uninfluenced by glucocorticoids, administration of these hormones induces the enzyme in the 1- to 12-day-old rat, but not in the fetal or adult animal, according to one report. As the animal ages beyond the suckling stage, there is a decrease in the concentration of the activating enzyme in liver. There is significant activating enzyme in the liver of the human fetus or premature infant at birth.

The transmethylase which acts upon the ethanolamines is at low concentration in the fetal rat liver, rises sharply at birth, then decreases gradually with growth to adulthood. Choline oxidase increases in level by 75 per cent in kidney as the rat develops from weaning stage to adult. Sarcosine dehydrogenase increases in level in rat liver beginning before birth and reaching a plateau at about 30 days. As rats age from the weaning stage (6 gm) to a weight of 280 gm, the betaine-homocysteine transmethylase content of liver decreases slightly on the basis of specific activity but shows no change on the basis of the whole organ. Over the same time period, the methyl-tetrahydrofolate-homocysteine transmethylase level decreases in liver, kidney, and brain, but increases in pancreas.

Rationalization of the regulation of the methionine-activating enzyme seems to be impossible at this time. No consistent pattern appears to emerge from the often contradictory reports on regulatory influences.

It seems reasonable that the reactions leading from the ethanolamines to choline should be favored in choline deficiency and that the reaction destroying choline (the oxidase) should be hindered under conditions of choline or methyl deficiency (or protein deficiency, which is one form of methyl deficiency). On the other hand, it seems metabolically inappropriate that choline oxidase be induced by high-fat diets, since choline-containing phospholipids are important factors in the synthesis of lipoproteins in the liver and the transport of lipid via these vehicles in the blood to the extrahepatic tissues (lipotropism). Increase in the level of choline oxidase in deficiency of vitamin B_{12} may be an adaptation to favor the production of betaine (a potential source of methionine methyl groups) when the cobamide-requiring pathway is hindered.

It is of interest to compare the effects of certain regulatory factors on the two transmethylase enzymes which regenerate methionine from homocysteine, the betaine and methyl-tetrahydrofolate enzymes, respectively. Some investigators are of the opinion that the betaine enzyme is concerned chiefly with the metabolism of betaine or homocysteine as such, whereas the function of the methyl-tetrahydrofolate enzyme is directly related to the need for resynthesis of methionine. This hypothesis is supported by several of the observed regulatory effects. Given that methionine is an essential amino acid, it is to be expected that the enzyme most concerned with its preservation (the methyl-tetrahydrofolate transmethylase) would be elevated in level on diets low in protein or in sulfur-containing amino acids, whereas such an enzyme might well be repressed by a high-protein diet or a load of methionine. It will be noted that many of these factors have exactly opposite effects on the betaine enzyme.

It seems metabolically appropriate that a key enzyme of *de novo* methyl group synthesis, methylene(formaldehyde)-tetrahydrofolate reductase, should be inhibited by S-adenosylmethionine, the chief agent of transmethylation, and that this inhibition should be relieved by the demethylated form of the agent, S-adenosylhomocysteine, thus neatly adapting the supply to the demand for methyl groups.

Granted all of the foregoing, there still remain many regulatory influences (as can be seen in Fig. 6-9) which cannot be explained at this time.

Polyamine Pathway (Fig. 6-10)

The diamine putrescine, and the polyamines spermidine and spermine are synthesized by a relatively straightforward sequence of reactions. Ornithine (derived from arginine) is decarboxylated to putrescine in a reaction requiring pyridoxal phosphate as coenzyme. To the resultant diaminobutane foundation are added, successively, a first and then a second propylamine moiety, leading to the formation of spermidine and spermine, respectively.

It may be recalled that, in discussing the activation of methionine in a previous section, it was pointed out that all three of the groups residing on the sulfonium pole of S-adenosylmethionine were endowed with considerable transfer potential, as was illustrated by various transfers of methyl groups, for one. Transfer of the carbon-nitrogen skeleton of

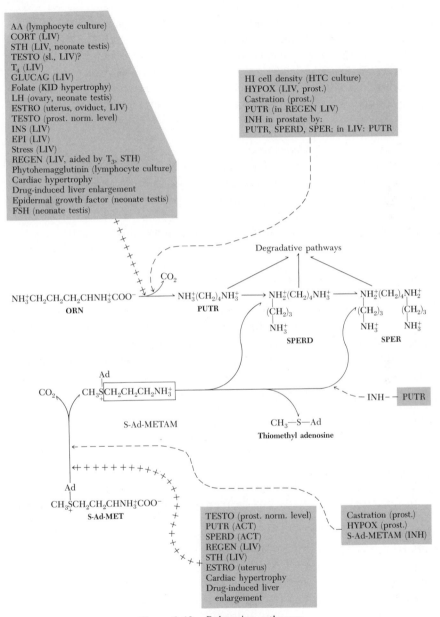

Figure 6–10.   Polyamine pathways.

methionine is an example of another, although it requires prior loss of the carboxyl group, the remaining propylamine moiety being that required for the synthesis of the polyamines.

In rat prostate gland, brain and liver and in yeast, the decarboxylation of S-adenosylmethionine and the subsequent transfers of the propylamine fragment are catalyzed by separate enzymes. The product of the decarboxylation goes under the rather awkward name of decarboxylated S-adenosylmethionine. By analogy with histamine, tyramine, and other amines derived from decarboxylation of amino acids, the amine arising from methionine should be called *methiamine,* and the compound in question in this pathway, *S-adenosylmethiamine.* Confusion with derivatives of thiamine should be minimal in most contexts.

There is evidence that, at least in rat liver, two propylamine transferases exist — spermidine synthase and spermine synthase. In either case, after loss of the propylamine group, the residue of thiomethyladenosine is degraded by phosphorylytic cleavage and subsequent reactions characteristic of pentose and purine metabolism.

Little is known of the degradative pathways of the polyamines. One enzyme which oxidizes spermidine and spermine is restricted in occurrence largely to the blood plasma of ruminants; the amine oxidase found in human plasma does not attack these two amines. It is probable, however, that appropriate amine oxidases exist in the mammal generally, since possible oxidation products are found in the organism. Thus, there occurs in brain a compound, putreanine, which has the structure of a spermidine molecule, the propylamine moiety of which has apparently been oxidatively deaminated (probably via the aldehyde) to a propionate group. Actually, diamine oxidase (histaminase) attacks not only the diamine, putrescine, but also the polyamines spermidine and spermine. The general catabolic sequence is, first, oxidative deamination of amino groups and formation of aldehydes and then further oxidation to carboxylic acids.

As is frequently the case in the specialized pathways discussed in this chapter, the regulation of polyamine synthesis is quite organ-specific. Thus, the ornithine decarboxylase level of liver is increased by growth hormone, glucocorticoids, thyroid hormones, testosterone (reported as slight by some, no effect by others), glucagon, estrogen, insulin, catecholamines, conditions of stress, liver regeneration, and liver enlargement caused by drugs. In other specialized situations, the enzyme is induced in cardiac hypertrophy, in kidney hypertrophy caused by folate administration, in the ovary by luteinizing hormone, in the uterus by estrogen, in the prostate by testosterone, in the testis of the neonate by follicle-stimulating, luteinizing, and growth hormones, and by epidermal growth factor, and in cultures of lymphocytes by stimulation with phytohemagglutinin. Addition of certain amino acids to the culture medium of lymphocytes induces the decarboxylase by repressing degradative reactions; glycine, serine, and asparagine are most effective.

Ornithine decarboxylase levels are reduced in the prostate by castration, in the prostate and liver by hypophysectomy, and in hepatoma cell cultures by high cell density. The rise in level after partial hepatectomy is blocked by injection of putrescine, suggesting the possible existence of control by product repression. Prostatic decarboxylase activity is competitively inhibited by putrescine, spermidine, and spermine, in the millimolar range, which may be physiologically realistic for the prostate. Putrescine also inhibits in liver.

S-Adenosylmethionine decarboxylase requires putrescine (or, less effectively, spermidine) as an activator. Many of the agents which induce ornithine decarboxylase do likewise in the case of the adenosylmethionine enzyme. Examples are testosterone in the prostate, estrogen in the uterus, growth hormone and regeneration in the liver, hypertrophy in the heart, and drug-mediated enlargement of the liver. Prostatic S-adenosylmethionine decarboxylase concentrations are reduced following castration or hypophysectomy. The prostatic enzyme is inhibited by one of the products, S-adenosylmethiamine.

Little is known of the regulation of the propylamine transferases. Spermine synthase of rat prostate and liver is inhibited by putrescine.

The temporal regulation of polyamine metabolism exhibits some noteworthy features. Ornithine decarboxylase, generally considered the rate-limiting enzyme in the synthetic sequence, has the shortest half-life of any mammalian enzyme thus far investigated. This turns out to be, under appropriate conditions in rat liver, of the order of 10 minutes.

In the rat, the ornithine decarboxylase level of the fetal placenta increases from day 13 to term, whereas that of the maternal placenta gradually decreases, so that at term most of the enzyme is in the fetal tissue. Since the distribution of diamine oxidase is just the reverse of this, it has been suggested that putrescine formed in the fetal placenta is oxidized in the maternal placenta.

A detailed developmental study has shown that ornithine decarboxylase reaches a peak in the rat uterine endometrium on days 8 to 9 and in the whole embryo on days 12 to 15, following which it decreases to low values before birth. S-adenosylmethionine decarboxylase levels reach a maximum in the rat embryo on day 11, then decrease sharply to a low level by day 13. Assays of individual embryonic tissues, which are practical no earlier than day 15, indicate that the two enzyme activities are already descending from their maxima at that time. Actual amine concentrations in the embryo reach a peak on day 13, 3 days before the peak in tissue RNA concentration. In addition, spermine concentration rises in most tissues just before birth, then subsides.

Spermidine concentration exhibits a circadian rhythm in mouse brain and liver, the maximum occurring in the middle of the night, or the dark period. This coincides with a peak in motor activity in this species. These observations undoubtedly relate to circadian rhythms in one or more of the enzymes responsible for synthesis of the polyamines.

Rat liver ornithine decarboxylase exhibits such a rhythm (peaking at about 8 P.M.), dependent primarily on the timing of the ingestion of food, specifically protein, and requiring for its occurrence the presence of intact pituitary and adrenal glands or the injection of growth hormone and glucocorticoid as replacements.

An impressively voluminous literature has already accumulated on the biological role of the polyamines. Data from many systems, including all living forms thus far investigated, lead to the general conclusion that polyamines are associated with growth. The exact nature of this association may be left to the future to unravel, but as a bare minimum of a clue, it is reasonably well established that polyamines participate in formation of ribosomes, maintenance of ribosomal integrity, or both. Thus, the connection of these compounds with conditions of increased protein synthesis is understandable.

Many of the regulatory factors previously listed for the two decarboxylases are exactly in accord with the foregoing remarks, such as the effects of various gonadotropic hormones upon their target tissues (in which protein synthesis and growth are promoted), and the effects of growth hormone and insulin on the liver. The influence of what are commonly considered protein-catabolic hormones is more difficult to explain, examples being the effects on liver of thyroid hormones, glucagon, glucocorticoids, and catecholamines. However, these substances, all of which are hepatotropic factors in the translocation of nitrogen in the organism, not only favor the transfer of amino acids from muscle to liver and increase the rate of gluconeogenesis in the liver but also favor the synthesis of a certain amount of hepatic and plasma protein.

There is no need to reiterate the observations connecting polyamines with development of the embryo. One final example of tissue growth may be mentioned: polyamine excretion in the urine of cancer patients is markedly increased over that of normal controls.

LYSINE: CARNITINE PATHWAY (Fig. 6-11)

Although it has been known for some time that butyrobetaine is a precursor of carnitine, lysine has been identified as the source of the former only recently. Evidently the epsilon amino group of lysine is successively methylated three times by S-adenosylmethionine to form the hypothetical intermediate, epsilon-N-trimethyllysine. From this point to the appearance of butyrobetaine the pathway is obscure. Carnitine is formed finally by oxidation of the betaine. A major catabolic pathway of carnitine is its decarboxylation to beta-methylcholine, an intramitochondrial reaction.

The overall rate of incorporation of labeled methyl groups from

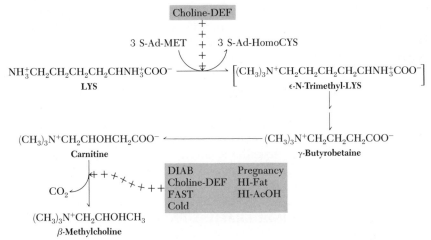

Figure 6–11. Carnitine pathway.

methionine into carnitine is increased in choline deficiency, although the incorporation into choline is accelerated to an even greater extent.

Decarboxylation of carnitine is increased in diabetes, pregnancy, fasting, cold-adaptation, high-fat diets, acetate loading, and in choline deficiency. Certain of these experimental conditions exhibit individual peculiarities. Thus, although both the diabetic state and cold-adaptation are characterized by increased conversion of carnitine to methylcholine and by a decreased half-life of carnitine (increased rate of turnover), the diabetic animal has a smaller total body pool and lower muscle concentration of carnitine, whereas acclimitization to cold results in increases in these two parameters.

Until the 1950's, the outstanding feature of carnitine was its requirement in insect nutrition, in which area it was known as vitamin B_T, after the mealworm, *Tenebrio molitor.* Since then, carnitine has become established as a significant factor in fatty acid metabolism in higher animals as well. Its role is that of a transport agent, carrying long-chain fatty acids from the cytosol into the mitochondria, which otherwise are impermeable to these metabolites or their CoA thioesters.

In view of its physiological function, it is interesting that all of the conditions in which the conversion of carnitine to beta-methylcholine is accelerated, except for choline deficiency, are characterized by an augmented rate of oxidation of fatty acids. This may seem surprising, since carnitine should be required in even greater amounts in such situations, whereas the decarboxylation is a means of intramitochondrial destruction of carnitine. However, the suggestion has been made that, during accelerated oxidation of fatty acids such large amounts of carnitine are brought into the organelle that perhaps carnitine would begin to compete for acyl, or more probably acetyl units, with those intramitochondrial systems involved in oxidation of acetate and other pathways of acetate metabolism. Hence, the decarboxylation pathway may serve as a disposal route for surplus carnitine.

It is not clear why a condition of choline deficiency should result in enhancement of the same pathway. However, since methyl-deficient diets generally cause some sort of compensatory augmentation in the rates of various transmethylation reactions, such as the synthesis of choline and of the hypothetical trimethyllysine precursor of carnitine, it is possible that simultaneous enhancement of a catabolic pathway represents a form of regulatory insurance against overproduction.

TRYPTOPHAN: INDOLEAMINE PATHWAY (Fig. 6-12)

The two indoleamines serotonin and melatonin share a common synthetic route, since the former is precursor of the latter. However, the synthesis of melatonin is confined to the pineal gland, whereas serotonin, in addition to the pineal, is formed in brain and in the enterochromaffin cells of the intestine.

Hydroxylation of the indole ring of tryptophan is the first, and probably rate-limiting step in serotonin synthesis. In most tissues where serotonin formation is significant in magnitude, this reaction is catalyzed by a specific tryptophan hydroxylase. In liver, the same reaction can be effected by phenylalanine hydroxylase, which has somewhat broader specificity than its name indicates. Liver, however, is not a major source of serotonin. The regulatory factors which will be discussed in connection with this hydroxylation reaction will be those influencing the "true" tryptophan hydroxylases.

The decarboxylase which converts hydroxytryptophan to hydroxytryptamine (serotonin) definitely is nonspecific. Wherever it occurs, it is a general arylamino acid decarboxylase, active upon indoleamino acids, catecholamino acids, and even (albeit feebly) imidazoleamino acids (histidine).

The major catabolic pathway of serotonin involves oxidative deamination of the side-chain amino group, forming the corresponding aldehyde, a reaction catalyzed by monoamine oxidase. Aldehyde dehydrogenases or oxidases then form hydroxyindoleacetate, which is excreted in the urine.

If the two steps required for formation of serotonin occur in the pineal gland, then two additional steps can lead to the production of melatonin: the action of serotonin N-acetyltransferase (acetylase), followed by the action of hydroxyindole-O-methyltransferase (O-methylase). The respective group donors are acetyl-CoA and S-adenosylmethionine. The acetylation is said to be rate-limiting under usual conditions.

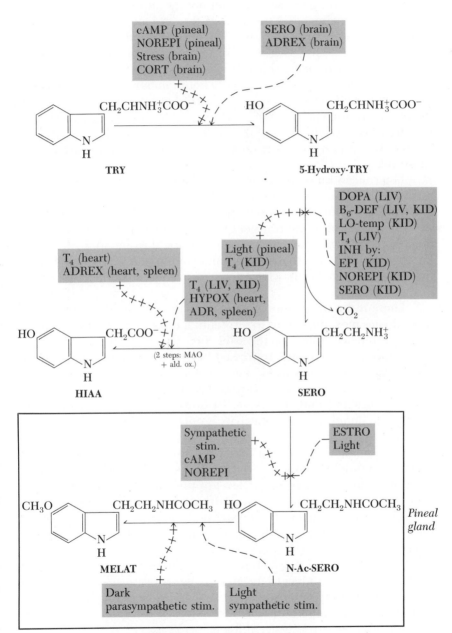

Figure 6–12. Indoleamine pathway.

The tryptophan hydroxylase level of the rat midbrain, which is lowered by adrenalectomy, is restored to normal by administration of glucocorticoids. In the normal rat, but not the adrenalectomized rat, exposure to stress also raises the level of this enzyme in brain. In the rat pineal gland in organ culture, the hydroxylase is induced by cAMP and norepinephrine. The hydroxylation *reaction* in brain appears to be under some type of negative feedback control from tissue levels of serotonin; since there is reason to exclude both inhibition and repression of the enzyme itself, it has been hypothesized that serotonin interferes with the transport of tryptophan into the brain. The substrate concentration may well be rate-limiting for the brain hydroxylase, since tryptophan levels in that organ are of the same order of magnitude as the K_m of the substrate.

The concentration of serotonin in the rat brain is elevated temporarily by administration of insulin or by feeding a meal of carbohydrate and thus stimulating insulin secretion. The elevation in brain serotonin probably is caused by the transient insulin-mediated elevation in plasma (and brain) tryptophan concentration, since this amino acid, for unknown reasons, reacts to insulin administration in a manner contrary to that of other amino acids, which decrease in concentration in the plasma in such circumstances.

There is no information on the regulation of the decarboxylase in those tissues most important to serotonin metabolism, other than the favorable influence of light on the level of enzyme in the pineal. In kidney, it is induced by thyroxine, repressed by exposure to low temperatures and by pyridoxine deficiency, and inhibited by serotonin and the catecholamines. The hepatic decarboxylase is repressed by DOPA, pyridoxine deficiency, and thyroxine. In human brain, the decarboxylase may be rate-limiting, since its activity is only 1/100 that of the analogous enzyme in rat brain.

Monoamine oxidase is an important factor in the disposal of serotonin, even in tissues in which the compound does not arise originally. Thyroid hormones increase the level of the oxidase in the heart of the young rat or in the adult female. Adrenalectomy does the same in the heart and spleen. Curiously, thyroid hormones repress the enzyme in the liver and kidney, as does hypophysectomy in the heart, adrenals, and spleen.

In the pineal gland, which not only synthesizes serotonin, but goes on to convert this product to melatonin, the acetylase enzyme is induced by cAMP and norepinephrine in organ culture, by sympathetic stimulation *in vivo*. Estrogen counteracts the effect of catecholamines *in vitro*, whereas light has a repressive influence *in vivo*.

The pineal O-methylase is induced rather weakly by cAMP and norepinephrine, the major inducers being darkness and parasympathetic (cholinergic) stimulation. The enzyme is repressed by light and sympathetic stimulation.

Tryptophan hydroxylase is present in significant concentration in the rat pineal gland at birth, increases to within 80 per cent of adult levels in the immediate postnatal period, and remains constant to about the twentieth day, when it rises to the adult level. The pineal decarboxylase level is very low until the twentieth postnatal day, then increases to day 30, remains constant to day 50, undergoes another increase to day 60, and then levels off. Pineal monoamine oxidase is absent at birth, increases very slightly for 2 weeks, and then increases more significantly to day 35, after which it levels off or increases slowly.

Rat brain tryptophan hydroxylase occurs in low concentration at birth (in brain stem, 30 per cent of adult; in cortex, 10 per cent of adult), and remains low for the first 10 postnatal days. A rapid rise then follows, reaching adult levels by about the twentieth day (stem) or thirtieth day (cortex).

Brain arylamino acid decarboxylase begins at a significant level in the late fetal period, increases to 70 per cent of the adult level by birth, also undergoes a temporary setback at birth or shortly thereafter, and then increases further. In the brain of the fetal rat, monoamine oxidase undergoes a spurt in concentration just before birth, reverses temporarily at birth, and then increases in the postnatal period to the time of weaning, when it levels off at adult values.

Monoamine oxidase in tissues other than pineal or brain also undergoes characteristic changes in level after birth. In liver, it increases during the first postnatal week, slows down by the second week, and then levels off until day 28, after which it gradually increases. In kidney there is no change in the low level for the first week, then a rise occurs during the second week, followed by a slower increase to day 42. Heart muscle shows practically no activity until the seventh postnatal day, then a slow increase to day 14, a sharp rise to day 28, a sharp drop to day 42, and then a slow increase. In the small intestine, monoamine oxidase levels decrease at birth from their already low values to practically zero in 1 week, increase sharply to day 14, decrease gradually to day 42, then increase very slowly.

The field of indoleamine metabolism provides several interesting examples of circadian rhythm. Although there is some disagreement in the literature as to the timing of the cycles, and although there are characteristic patterns in the individual regions of the brain, most reports agree that the concentration of serotonin in rat brain reaches a maximum during the daylight (or artificial light) hours and a minimum during the dark.

In the rat pineal gland, the concentrations of serotonin and melatonin exhibit circadian rhythms which are inverse to each other, although both ultimately utilize the lighting schedule as *Zeitgeber*. In the adult rat, perception of light by the retina results in sympathetic stimulation of the pineal gland, inducing the decarboxylase and leading to a peak in serotonin concentration during the daylight hours. The concentration falls to a minimum in the dark period. The rhythm is not abolished by blinding the suckling rat, in which the harderian gland functions as phototransducer. It is reported also that the young rat differs from the mature in that the rhythm is retained after destruction of sympathetic innervation of the gland.

On the other hand, exposure to light results in repression of the acetylase and O-methylase in the rat pineal. As in the previous case, the harderian gland can replace the retina as photoreceptor in the suckling rat. Melatonin concentration in the pineal gland thus declines to a minimum in the light period and rises to a maximum in the dark. This last phase is not passive, since the O-methylase has been shown to be induced by parasympathetic stimulation triggered by darkness. It is interesting that the varying concentrations of the enzymes with time cause the acetylase to be rate-limiting during the day, whereas the O-methylase is the less active during the night.

Rat pineal serotonin acetylase is detectable in the fetus 4 days before birth. Traces of a circadian rhythm appear on the fourth postnatal day. Around the seventh day, the daylight level drops to one-half to one-third that at birth, while the nocturnal level continues to climb until it reaches adult values in the third postnatal week. The sensitivity of the enzyme to induction by norepinephrine is established by the third postnatal day and increases rapidly thereafter.

It is difficult, perhaps almost impossible at this time, to rationalize the regulatory factors in the metabolism of serotonin and melatonin, since the physiological functions of neither compound have been well established in the mammal. It is believed by some that serotonin plays a role in the control of sleep. It is interesting, therefore, that the peak in concentration of serotonin in the brain of the rat occurs in daylight, when this rodent is asleep or at least quiescent. However, if this relationship is valid, then it is difficult to explain the induction of the hydroxylase by stress and glucocorticoids in the brain and by catecholamines in the pineal.

In the amphibian and some other cold-blooded animals, melatonin has an important function in the adaptation of the skin color of the animal to that of its surroundings, by causing aggregation of melanin and thus lightening of the skin color, in opposition to the melanin-dispersing influence of the melanocyte-stimulating hormones. The role of melatonin in the mammal is very uncertain, although antigonadotropic properties have been demonstrated. If these properties are true physiological functions of the compound, and if one assumes that gonadal activity is largely a nocturnal affair in the rodent, then the circadian cycle of melatonin makes sense.

Of the other regulatory influences found in this metabolic pathway, the feedback controls seem reasonable, as they usually do, and many of the developmental controls appear appropriate, in the sense that they indicate spurts of enzyme synthesis either at birth or at weaning, when new and more complex patterns of behavior may well require the presence of certain neurohormones in the brain or pineal gland.

TYROSINE

Thyroxine Pathway (Fig. 6–13)

The synthesis of thyroid hormones begins with the active uptake by the thyroid gland of the inorganic iodide derived from the diet (and from the previous catabolism of iodinated compounds in the body). A peroxidase then oxidizes the iodide to iodine, which is utilized in the iodination of tyrosine and its derivatives. Protein-bound (thyroglobulin or its precursors) residues of tyrosine are converted first to monoiodotyrosine (MIT), then to diiodotyrosine (DIT) residues. A coupling process between two residues of DIT or between one residue each of MIT and DIT then produces thyroxine (T_4) or triiodothyronine (T_3), respectively. The iodinated thyroglobulin, which is located in the follicles of the gland, is digested by a thyroidal protease, releasing the iodinated derivatives, chiefly T_4 and T_3, into the bloodstream.

Although the pharmacology of the thyroid has been investigated very actively, at least with respect to the search for active analogs of the hormones and for inhibitors of the various steps in the synthetic pathway, little is known of the physiological control of the system. Each step in the sequence appears to be accelerated by the thyrotropic hormone (thyroid-stimulating hormone, TSH) of the anterior pituitary, the secretion of which is controlled by a hypothalamic releasing factor (TRF). All of the effects of TSH upon the thyroid gland are believed to be mediated by cAMP. Free T_4 and T_3 form part of a negative feedback system, the thyroid hormones in circulation depressing the stimuli for their own formation by inhibition of the secretion of TRF at the hypothalamic level and of TSH at the pituitary level.

The iodination reaction catalyzed by thyroidal peroxidase is inhibited *in vitro* by glutathione at 5×10^{-5} M, but it is not known if this effect is physiological.

In addition to their spectacular role in amphibian metamorphosis, the thyroid hormones appear to be particularly important in the development of the nervous system, skeleton, and skin of the mammal. The thyroid gland becomes functional at varying times in different mammals, occurring at the late fetal stage in rats, at which time, as has been noted elsewhere, the thyroid hormones induce certain of the enzymes of amino acid metabolism.

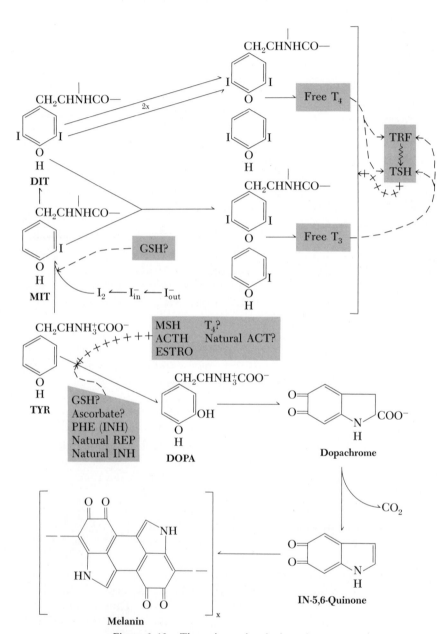

Figure 6–13. Thyroxine and melanin pathways.

Melanin Pathway (Fig. 6-13)

The synthesis of melanin differs from most other pathways in that it is dependent upon the activity of only one enzyme, tyrosinase. This copper-containing enzyme is characterized by the possession of two catalytic activities, a monophenolase or hydroxylase, plus a catecholase or diphenolase, the action of the latter resulting in the formation of unstable intermediates of the orthoquinone type. The mixture of mono- and polyphenols and quinones can undergo such a variety of interactions that it is impossible to state where the action of the enzyme ceases and autocatalytic reactions take over.

Taking the oversimplified scheme of Figure 6-13 as a first approximation, tyrosine is oxidized by tyrosinase in organelles called *melanosomes* within cells called *melanocytes*, forming initially dihydroxyphenylalanine (DOPA), which itself has an autocatalytic effect on this first reaction. DOPA is oxidized further in several steps to form dopachrome, which is decarboxylated to indolequinone. Condensation of many molecules of the quinone forms the highly polymeric melanin, which may exist in a more reduced (brown) or in a more oxidized form (black, as shown in the figure). In the skin, the melanosomes, charged with melanin, may be transferred, via the dendritic processes of the melanocytes, to the nearby keratinocytes (malpighian cells), where they impart the appropriate degree of darkening to the skin.

Epidermal melanogenesis is induced in mammals by estrogens, possibly thyroid hormones, and by any of a family of pituitary polypeptide hormones called melanocyte-stimulating hormones (MSH). ACTH has similar activity, apparently due to appreciable homology in amino acid sequence. Release of MSH from the pituitary is controlled by an inhibitor (MIH) from the hypothalamus. Melatonin and glucocorticoids also inhibit release, possibly functioning via MIH. There is some evidence that tyrosinase is synthesized initially as an inactive protyrosinase, which is activated in the melanosomes by as yet unidentified natural activators.

Synthesis of tyrosinase is repressed by unidentified natural substances. Its activity is inhibited by similarly unidentified substances, some containing sulfhydryl groups (glutathione?), by naturally occurring reductants such as ascorbate, and by phenylalanine, the effect of which requires only slightly supranormal concentrations. This last observation has been invoked as an explanation of the light coloration usually encountered in phenylketonurics, who have elevated concentrations of phenylalanine in the blood if untreated.

Although epidermal melanin in mammals is not subject to the same type of controls over its state of aggregation or dispersion found in certain other forms of life, it is of considerable interest, and may represent some sort of evolutionary vestige, that MSH does promote the transport of melanin granules through the dendritic processes of the melanocytes to the overlying keratinocytes, resulting in a general darkening effect.

Since further analogies may be found in the future, it may be worthwhile to mention at this point that, in the amphibian skin, aggregation of melanin (resulting in lightening) is favored by melatonin, catecholamines, and acetylcholine, whereas dispersion (darkening) is favored by MSH and by agents (such as caffeine) which stimulate synthesis of cAMP.

In the skin of the fetal hamster, tyrosinase levels increase smoothly from the fourteenth fetal day to the sixth postnatal day, after which a plateau is established. Around day 16 the enzyme level decreases until, by day 22, it is at the level of the first or second postnatal day, after which the level remains constant at least to day 32. In brown and black mice, after the postnatal maximum, there occurs a decline to zero detectable activity, whereas in the black rat, the generally similar pattern is terminated by a decrease to low, but not negligible, levels.

Catecholamine Pathway (Fig. 6-14)

Three compounds are included in the category of catecholamines: dihydroxyphenylethylamine (dopamine), norepinephrine, and epinephrine. Although connected in a metabolic sequence in the order given, each amine is not merely a precursor or product of another, but rather is endowed with its own physiological functions. Dopamine, for example, seems to play an important, but at present not well clarified, role in the central nervous system, since it is present in subnormal concentration in the brain of patients afflicted with parkinsonism, the symptoms of which can be ameliorated by administration of DOPA (dihydroxyphenylalanine), which is taken up by the brain and converted to dopamine. Norepinephrine is the neurotransmitter of sympathetic nerve endings, functioning at the local level, whereas epinephrine, synthesized primarily by the adrenal medulla, behaves like a classic hormone by being secreted into the general circulation for action elsewhere.

As might be anticipated, catecholamines are synthesized mainly in the central nervous system, peripheral sympathetic nerves, and the adrenal medulla, with small amounts arising also in chromaffin cells, which are distributed in various parts of the body. Intracellularly, catecholamines are found in storage granules. Their uptake into and release from these granules are processes which are currently under intensive investigation.

Synthesis of the catecholamines begins with the conversion of tyrosine to DOPA, considered the rate-limiting reaction of the entire sequence, and catalyzed by tyrosine hydroxylase. A pteridine cofactor is required (cf. phenylalanine hydroxylase). DOPA is decarboxylated by the general arylamino acid decarboxylase to dopamine, which is converted to norepinephrine by dopamine beta-hydroxylase. Although traces of epinephrine are formed elsewhere, it is chiefly in the adrenal medulla where norepinephrine is methylated to epinephrine under the influence of phenylethanolamine N-methyltransferase.

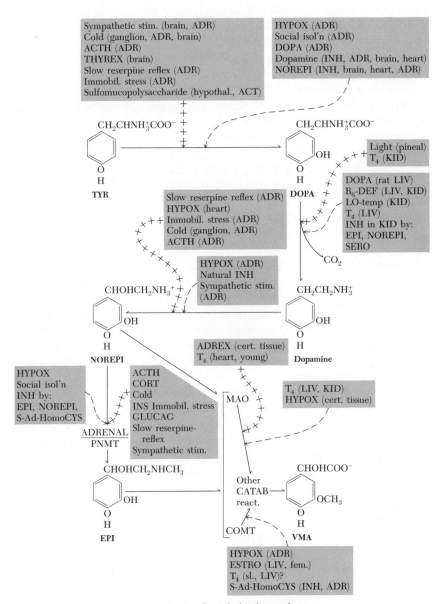

Figure 6–14. Catecholamine pathway.

The nature of the catabolic pathway followed by the catecholamines depends to some extent upon where they happen to be found. If, for example, norepinephrine is liberated at a sympathetic synapse, its major route of disappearance will not be catabolic at all, but will be primarily a matter of re-uptake into storage granules. Within the nerve cells proper, the major true degradative route involves oxidation by monoamine oxidase, whereas catecholamines in the general circulation are subject to both oxidation by monoamine oxidase and O-methylation (catecholamine O-methyltransferase, COMT) in the extraneural tissues. Since there is no information available on regulation of catabolic reactions other than these two, further details of the catabolic route will be omitted. It will suffice to point out that the major excretory product of catecholamine catabolism is methoxyhydroxymandelate, *vanilmandelate.*

Adrenal medullary tyrosine hydroxylase activity is elevated rapidly by sympathetic stimulation, more gradually by reflexive stimulation due to prolonged administration of reserpine. The former effect is one of activation by removal of an inhibitor, norepinephrine, through rapid discharge from the gland; the latter apparently represents true induction of *de novo* synthesis of the enzyme. Administration of ACTH maintains normal, but does not induce supernormal, levels of the enzyme in the adrenals of hypophysectomized rats. The adrenal enzyme is induced by immobilization stress and by cold (which also induces the enzyme in the superior cervical ganglion and in the medulla of the brain). Thyroidectomy and sympathetic stimulation increase the concentration of the hydroxylase in brain. A purified preparation of the enzyme from the canine hypothalamus is activated by sulfated mucopolysaccharides, which may have some connection with the association of the enzyme with membranous structures in the nervous system *in vivo.*

Hypophysectomy, social isolation, and large doses of DOPA decrease the level of tyrosine hydroxylase in the adrenal. In brain, heart, and adrenals, the activity of the enzyme is inhibited by norepinephrine (also, reportedly, by dopamine), which competes with the pteridine cofactor. Tyrosine hydroxylase of bovine adrenal medulla and brain is inhibited by high levels of oxygen, possibly accounting for the neurotoxic effects of high concentrations of oxygen in the newborn, and for the decrease in brain norepinephrine and dopamine and in heart norepinephrine in animals exposed to hyperbaric oxygen.

Hyperthyroidism in rats and guinea pigs results in increased concentration of the arylamino acid decarboxylase in kidney, but the converse change in liver. The pineal decarboxylase is induced by exposure of the animal to light. Exposure to low temperatures (or the winter season) lowers the level of this enzyme in guinea pig kidney. Avitaminosis B_6 decreases the activity of the decarboxylase in both liver and kidney of the rat; since only the kidney activity is restored by pyridoxal phosphate *in vitro,* the effect in liver must be caused by an actual decrease in apoenzyme. Large doses of DOPA cause a drop in decarboxylase level in rat liver but not in any of several other tissues tested. Epinephrine, norepinephrine, and serotonin inhibit the renal decarboxylase. In contrast to the situation in the rat, the specific activity of the decarboxylase of human brain is so low that it, rather than the tyrosine hydroxylase, may be rate-limiting.

The response of the adrenal dopamine beta-hydroxylase toward neural stimulation is rather odd. Although the slow response to prolonged stimulation resembles that of tyrosine hydroxylase, the short-term reaction to more direct sympathetic stimulation is first a decrease in activity of the enzyme, and only somewhat later an increase. The level of the beta-hydroxylase also is raised in the adrenal by immobilization stress and exposure to cold (which has the same effect in various ganglia), and in the heart by hypophysectomy. It is noteworthy that, in the adrenal, hypophysectomy decreases the level of the enzyme, which can be restored only partly by administration of ACTH. Natural inhibitors of the hydroxylase occur in many tissues of the rat. One which has been purified from heart contains carbohydrate, phosphate, and a trace of nitrogen, and is believed to function by chelation of the cupric ion cofactor of the enzyme. Another, from the adrenal, is a peptide resembling but not identical with glutathione.

The adrenal phenylethanolamine N-methyltransferase, which is decreased in level by hypophysectomy, is restored to normal values by either ACTH or glucocorticoids. It can be raised to above-normal levels by the rapid sympathetic stimulation or the slower reserpine treatment mentioned earlier, and by any of various forms of stress (immobilization, exposure to cold, injection of insulin or glucagon).

In addition to hypophysectomy, the level of the transmethylase in the adrenal also can be lowered by social isolation. Its activity is inhibited by epinephrine (and reportedly by norepinephrine) and by S-adenosylhomocysteine, one of the products of the transmethylation.

On the catabolic side, monoamine oxidase is induced by adrenalectomy in rat heart, spleen, superior cervical ganglion, hypothalamus, and vas deferens, but not in other areas of the brain, liver, or kidney. Thyroid hormones increase the level of the oxidase in the heart of the young female rat. In contrast, although certain early publications made claims to the contrary, recent reports agree that, in liver and kidney, thyroid hormones lower the level of monoamine oxidase in rat and rabbit. Hypophysectomy has the same effect in rat heart, spleen, hypothalamus, kidney, and adrenal, but not in liver or several other tissues.

Catechol O-methyltransferase may be slightly repressed by thyroid hormones in rat liver, but is definitely repressed by estrogen in the liver of the female rat and by hypophysectomy in the adrenal. The enzyme is inhibited by S-adenosylhomocysteine.

It is not certain at this time exactly how the uptake and release of catecholamines from storage granules fits into the general regulatory picture, although an instance of the participation of neural release mechanisms in this regulation has been cited already. Uptake is favored by the presence of ATP, magnesium ions, and sodium ions (cf. requirements for active transport of amino acids) and is blocked by tyramine, a phenolamine formed by decarboxylation of tyrosine and usually accompanying the catecholamines in nature. Release is promoted by acetylcholine, calcium ions, neural stimulation, and tyramine, and is blocked by the prostaglandins.

In the brain of the newborn rat, which has poor functional development at that time, levels of norepinephrine and monoamine oxidase are low. The guinea pig, which is functionally well developed when born, has almost adult levels of the amine and oxidase in its brain. It should be noted, however, that the situation is not entirely so simple, since the newborn rat brain contains nearly adult levels of arylamino acid decarboxylase.

Injection of nerve growth factor into newborn rats induces tyrosine hydroxylase and dopamine beta-hydroxylase in the superior cervical ganglion. In the course of normal development, tyrosine hydroxylase is present in rat brain on the fifteenth day of gestation, but increases greatly in level with maturation, during which there is also a shift in location of the enzyme from the soluble phase to the *synaptosome* fraction (nerve terminals sheared off during homogenization). Dopamine beta-hydroxylase follows the same general pattern, increasing from the fifteenth day in a slightly sigmoid curve to the adult level, simultaneously shifting to the synaptosome fraction, and also increasing more rapidly in the rostral than in the caudal regions of the brain.

The N-methyltransferase of the rat adrenal increases rapidly in the fetus, beginning about the eighteenth day, followed by accumulation of epinephrine. Both phenomena are blocked by removal of the influence of the pituitary (decapitation of the fetus), an effect reversed by administration of ACTH or glucocorticoids.

Monoamine oxidase, already mentioned as being present in only small amounts in the brain of the newborn rat, undergoes only slow development for the first 10 postnatal days, then its increase in level accelerates. In the adult rat, the half-life of monoamine oxidase is 4 to 6 days in submandibular gland, 4 days in liver, 10 to 13 days in heart, and 9 to 11 days in brain.

Rat pineal gland norepinephrine metabolism is characterized by a circadian rhythm resembling that of melatonin. Tyrosine hydroxylase concentration reaches a maximum in the dark period and a minimum in the light period.

If we accept the hypothesis of the Cannonical school of physiologists, that the function of the catecholamines (and of the sympathetic nervous system in general) is to prepare the organism for "fight or flight" in moments of danger, then many of the regulatory factors mentioned in the preceding discussion make metabolic sense. Biochemical and physiological effects of the catecholamines which would be useful in emergencies include

1. increase in the rate of glycogenolysis and gluconeogenesis in the liver, furnishing an increased supply of blood glucose, coupled with

2. inhibition of the glucose-stimulated release of insulin from the pancreas, thus favoring the uptake of glucose by the central nervous system rather than by other tissues;

3. increase in the rate of lipolysis in adipose tissue, furnishing an increased supply of free fatty acids to the circulation and thus supplying fuel for many extra-adipose tissues, e.g., muscle;

4. increase in the rate of glycogenolysis in skeletal muscle to lactate, providing another source of energy for muscle contraction, and, via the liver and Cori cycle, an additional source of blood glucose; and

5. various physiological adjustments, only one of which will be noted here as an example—increase in the force and rate of contraction of cardiac muscle.

It is evident that many of the factors which induce the catecholamine-synthesizing enzymes fit neatly into the preceding scheme. It is also evident that most of the instances of product or metabolite inhibition appear to be functioning as might be expected. On the other hand, it is difficult to see why thyroid hormones should have opposite effects on the decarboxylase in liver and kidney, and on monoamine oxidase in liver and heart. In the latter connection, it is altogether odd that hyperthyroidism results in repression of monoamine oxidase in the liver, since a catabolic and detoxifying enzyme might be expected to be utilized even to a greater extent in a condition of intensified metabolism.

CONCLUSIONS

Although perhaps not as obviously vital to the organism as those metabolic routes catalogued as ergogenic, the specialized amino acid pathways discussed in this chapter play their own essential roles in a less spectacular, and, it must be confessed, sometimes rather obscure manner. Nevertheless, each pathway, when investigated, has proved to be endowed with regulatory mechanisms which, in many cases, appear to be appropriately operative in adapting that reaction to its physiological role. The phrase "in many cases" is used advisedly, since more than a few instances have been noted in which, at the present time at least, no rationale whatever can be attributed to certain regulatory factors.

REFERENCES

Cysteine

Langdon, R. G., and Mize, C. E.: Recent studies on a mechanism of action of insulin. Bull. Johns Hopkins Hosp. *108*:146–148 (1961).
Horiuchi, K.: Experimental isovalthinuria–induction by hormones. Clin. Chim. Acta *12*:325–329 (1965).
Jacobsen, J. G., and Smith, L. H., Jr.: Biochemistry and physiology of taurine and taurine derivatives, Physiol. Rev. *48*:424–511 (1968).
Jackson, R. C.: Studies in the enzymology of glutathione metabolism in human erythrocytes. Biochem. J. *111*:309–315 (1969).
Little, C., Olinescu, R., Reid, K. G., and O'Brien, P. J.: Properties and regulation of glutathione peroxidase. J. Biol. Chem. *245*:3632–3636 (1970).

Glycine

Hartman, S. C.: Purines and pyrimidines. *In*: Greenberg, D. M. (ed.): Metabolic Pathways. Vol. 4. New York, Academic Press, Inc., 1970, pp. 1–68.
Kaplan, B. H.: The control of heme synthesis. *In*: Gordon, A. S. (ed.): Regulation of Hematopoiesis. Vol. 1. New York, Appleton-Century-Crofts, 1970, pp. 677–700.
Bank, A., Rifkind, R. A., and Marks, P. A.: Regulation of globin synthesis. *In*: Gordon, A. S. (ed.): Regulation of Hematopoiesis. Vol. 1. New York, Appleton-Century-Crofts, 1970, pp. 701–729.
Granick, S., and Sassa, S.: delta-Aminolevulinic acid synthetase and the control of heme and chlorophyll synthesis. *In*: Vogel, H. J. (ed.): Metabolic Pathways. Vol. 5. New York, Academic Press, Inc., 1971, pp. 77–141.
Marks, P. A., and Rifkind, R. A.: Protein synthesis: its control in erythropoiesis. Science *175*:955–961 (1972).

Glutamate

Baxter, C. F.: The nature of gamma-aminobutyric acid. *In*: Lajtha, A. (ed.): Handbook of Neurochemistry. Vol. 3. New York, Plenum Press, 1970, pp. 289–353.
van den Berg, C. J.: Glutamate and glutamine. *In*: Lajtha, A. (ed.): Handbook of Neurochemistry. Vol. 3. New York, Plenum Press, 1970, pp. 355–379.
Patterson, M. K., Jr., and Orr, G. R.: Asparagine synthesis by the Novikoff hepatoma. J. Biol. Chem. *243*:376–380 (1968).
Patterson, M. K., Jr., and Orr, G. R.: Regeneration, tumor, dietary, and L-asparagine effects on asparagine biosynthesis in rat liver. Cancer Res. *29*:1179–1183 (1969).
Hartman, S. C.: Purines and pyrimidines. *In*: Greenberg, D. M. (ed.): Metabolic Pathways. Vol. 4. New York, Academic Press, Inc., 1970, pp. 1–68.
Berlinguet, L., and Laliberté, M.: Biosynthesis of N-acetyl-L-aspartic acid in vivo and in brain homogenates. Can. J. Biochem. *48*:207–211 (1970).
Woods, J. S., and Handschumacher, R. E.: Hepatic homeostasis of plasma L-asparagine. Am. J. Physiol. *221*:1785–1790 (1971).

Arginine

Walker, J. B.: End-product repression in the creatine pathway of the developing chick embryo. Adv. Enz. Reg. *1*:151–168 (1963).
Ramírez, O., Calva, E., and Trejo, A.: Creatine regulation in the embryo and growing chick. Biochem. J. *119*:757–763 (1970).
Koszalka, T. R., Jensh, R., and Brent, R. L.: Creatine metabolism in the developing rat fetus. Comp. Biochem. Physiol. *41B*:217–229 (1972).

Histidine

Kapeller-Adler, R.: Amine Oxidases and Methods for their Study. New York, Wiley-Interscience, 1970, Chapter 4.

Kahlson, G., and Rosengren, E.: Biogenesis and Physiology of Histamine. London, Edward Arnold (Publishers) Ltd., 1971.

Stifel, F. B., and Herman, R. H.: Histidine metabolism. Am. J. Clin. Nutr. *24*:207–217 (1971).

Proline and Lysine (Collagen)

Kivirikko, K. I.: Hydroxyproline-containing fractions in normal and cortisone-treated chick embryos. Acta Physiol. Scand. *60*:suppl. 219 (1963). Review of the literature, pp. 9-21.

Houck, J. C., Sharma, V. K., and Carillo, A. L.: Control of cutaneous collagenolysis. Adv. Enz. Reg. *8*:269–278 (1970).

Grant, M. E., and Prockop, D. J.: The biosynthesis of collagen (in three parts). New Engl. J. Med. *286*:194–199, 242–249, 291–300 (1972).

Methionine

Lombardini, J. L., and Talalay, P.: Formation, functions, and regulatory importance of S-adenosyl-L-methionine. Adv. Enz. Reg. *9*:349–384 (1971).

Finkelstein, J. D., Kyle, W. E., and Harris, B. J.: Methionine metabolism in mammals. Regulation of homocysteine methyltransferases in rat tissues. Arch. Biochem. Biophys. *146*:84–92 (1971).

Kutzbach, C., and Stokstad, E. L. R.: Mammalian methylenetetrahydrofolate reductase. Biochim. Biophys. Acta *250*:459–477 (1971).

Cohen, S. S.: Introduction to the Polyamines. Englewood Cliffs, N. J., Prentice-Hall, Inc., 1971.

Williams-Ashman, H. G.: Control mechanisms in the biosynthesis of aliphatic amines in eukaryotic cells. *In*: Kun, E., and Grisolia, S. (eds.): Biochemical Regulatory Mechanisms in Eukaryotic Cells. New York, Wiley-Interscience, 1972, pp. 245–269.

Lysine (Carnitine)

Therriault, D. G., and Mehlman, M. A.: Metabolism of carnitine in cold-acclimated rats. Can. J. Biochem. *43*:1437–1443 (1965).

Khairallah, E. A., and Wolf, G.: Carnitine decarboxylase J. Biol. Chem. *242*:32–39 (1967).

Anon.; Choline deficiency and carnitine depletion. Nutr. Rev. *26*:152–154 (1968).

Mehlman, M. A., Kader, M. M. A., and Therriault, D. G.: Metabolism, turnover time, half life, body pool of carnitine-^{14}C in normal, alloxan diabetic and insulin treated rats. Life Sci. *8*(II):465–472 (1969).

Tryptophan

Black, I. B., and Axelrod, J.: The regulation of some biochemical circadian rhythms. *In*: Litwack, G. (ed.): Biochemical Actions of Hormones. Vol. 1. New York, Academic Press, Inc., 1970, pp. 135–155.

Weiss, B.: On the regulation of adenyl cyclase activity in the rat pineal gland. Ann. N. Y. Acad. Sci. *185*:507–519 (1971).

Tyrosine

Snell, R. S.: Hormonal control of pigmentation in man and other mammals. *In*: Montagna, W., and Hu, F. (eds.): Advances in Biology of Skin. Vol. 8. The Pigmentary System. New York, Pergamon Press, 1967, pp. 447–466.

Schell-Frederick, E., and Dumont, J. E.: Mechanism of action of thyrotropin. *In*: Litwack, G. (ed.): Biochemical Actions of Hormones. Vol. 1. New York, Academic Press, Inc., 1970, pp. 415–463.

Kapeller-Adler, R.: Amine Oxidases and Methods for their Study. New York, Wiley-Interscience, 1970, Chapter 3.

Molinoff, P. B., and Axelrod, J.: Biochemistry of the catecholamines. Ann. Rev. Biochem. *40*:465–500 (1971).

INDEX

"A" transport system, 37

Acetate, effect on carnitine metabolism, 173

Acetoneogenesis, 53

N-Acetylaspartate, pathway, 149

Acetylcholine, effect on catecholamine storage, 186

Acetyl-coenzyme A, effect on carbohydrate metabolism, 55

N-Acetylglutamate, effect on glutaminase, 131–132

effect on ornithine cycle, 121, 126

Acidosis, ammonia production, 131

effect on L-amino acid oxidase, 131

effect on gluconeogenesis, 133

effect on glutaminase, 131–132

effect on glutamine synthesis in liver, 130

effect on glutamine-ketoacid transaminase, 131

effect on glycine oxidase, 131

effect on pentose shunt pathway, 128

effect on renal hypertrophy, 128

effect on renal uptake of glutamine, 130

Acrasin, 13

Actinomycin-D, effect on tryptophan pyrrolase induction, 102

effect on tyrosine transaminase, 113, 115

in regulatory investigations, 9

"paradoxical" action, 105

sites of action, 9

Activation, definition, 2

Active transport, 35

Acute controls, 2

Adenosine diphosphate, effect on glutamine synthesis in liver, 130

effect on glutathione synthesis, 137

Adenosine triphosphate, effect on aminobutyrate pathway, 147

effect on branched-chain amino acid catabolism, 97

effect on catecholamine storage, 186

effect on glutathione peroxidase, 139

effect on Krebs cycle, 55

effect on proline synthesis, 90

S-Adenosylhomocysteine, effect on catechol O-methyltransferase, 185

effect on methyl group synthesis, 167

effect on one-carbon unit metabolism, 166

S-Adenosylhomocysteine (*Continued*)

effect on phenylethanolamine N-methyltransferase, 185

effect on S-adenosylmethionine decarboxylase, 171

S-Adenosylmethionine, decarboxylase, 171

effect on one-carbon unit metabolism, 166

synthesis, 163

Adenylate, as source of ammonia in muscle, 25–26

Adrenalectomy, effect on aminobutyrate pathway, 147

effect on blood level of diamine oxidase, 158

effect on branched-chain amino acid catabolism, 96

effect on glutamate dehydrogenase, 61

effect on glutamine synthesis in liver, 130

effect on glycine catabolism, 77

effect on histidine catabolism, 85, 87, 88

effect on monoamine oxidase, 176, 185

effect on ornithine cycle, 126

effect on proline catabolism, 90

effect on serine catabolism, 75

effect on serine synthesis, 73

effect on tryptophan catabolism, 102

effect on tryptophan hydroxylase, 176

Adrenocorticotropic hormone, effect on dopamine beta-hydroxylase, 185

effect on fat metabolism, 55

effect on histidine catabolism, 87

effect on isovalthine excretion, 139

effect on melanin synthesis, 181

effect on phenylethanolamine N-methyltransferase, 185

effect on transport of amino acids, 48

effect on tyrosine hydroxylase, 184

Age, effect on collagen synthesis, 161

Alanine, as major glucogenic amino acid, 60

effect on glutamine synthesis in brain, 145

in portal blood, 22

metabolism, regulation, 65

transport in diaphragm, 45

β-Alanine, effect on glutamine synthesis in liver, 130

Alanine cycle, 67

Alanine transaminase, development, 66
  regulation, 65
  role as regulator of gluconeogenesis,
    66–67
Alanine-preferring transport system, 37
Alkalosis, effect on excretion of citrate
  and ketoglutarate, 128
Allosteric effects, 6
Allylisopropylacetamide, 142
Allysine, 161
Amine oxidases. See also *Monoamine
  oxidase; Diamine oxidase.*
  effect on polyamines, 170
Amino acid(s), activation for protein
    synthesis, 3
  branched-chain, degradation in muscle,
    24–25
    extrahepatic degradation, 23
  catabolism, factors favoring, 30
  deamination, by intestinal bacteria, 22
    in liver, 22
  deposition in muscle, factors favoring, 29
  effect on branched-chain amino acid
    catabolism, 97
  effect on glycine catabolism, 77
  effect on histidine catabolism, 87, 88
  effect on ornithine decarboxylase, 170
  effect on ornithine transaminase, 83
  effect on serine catabolism, 74
  effect on tyrosine catabolism, 112
  essential, degradation in liver, 23
  glucogenic, definition, 52
  ketogenic, definition, 52
  metabolism, in gastrointestinal tract,
    20–22
  nonessential, degradation in muscle, 24
    synthesis in liver, 22
  supply, as regulatory factor, 60
  translocation, 27–29
  transport groups, 36
D-Amino acid oxidase, 58
L-Amino acid oxidase, 58
  in acidosis, 131
γ-Aminobutyrate, effect on aminobutyrate
    pathway, 147
  in brain, development, 148
  transaminase, 147
1-Aminocyclopentane-1-carboxylate, as
  model amino acid for transport, 38. See
  also *Cycloleucine.*
α-Aminoisobutyrate, as model amino acid
  for transport, 38
Aminolevulinate, dehydratase, 141
  synthase, 141
Aminooxyacetate, effect on aminobutyrate
  pathway, 148
β-Amino transport group, 38
Ammonia, as carrier of urinary hydrogen
    ions, 128
  detoxication in liver, 24

Ammonia (*Continued*)
  excretion, 26
  formation by intestinal bacteria, 22
  from adenylate in muscle, 25–26
  in portal blood, 22, 24
  sources in acidosis, 131
Amphibolic reactions, definition, 80
Anabolic pathways, regulation, 16
Anaphylactic shock, effect on blood level of
    diamine oxidase, 158
Anaplerotic reactions, definition, 80
Androgens. See *Testosterone.*
Anemia, effect on hemoglobin synthesis,
    145
Anionic transport group, 38
Anserine, in muscle, 26
Anticodon, 3
Arginase, 123
  rate of degradation as regulatory
    influence, 126
  regulation of, 82
Arginine, anabolic and catabolic pathways,
    80
  creatine pathway, 153
  effect on N-acetylglutamate synthesis, 121
  effect on arginase, 82
  effect on creatine synthesis, 154
  effect on ornithine cycle, 126
  effect on ornithine transaminase, 83, 84
Arginine-glycine transamidinase, 153–154
Argininosuccinate, lyase, 121
  synthetase, 121
Arylamino acid decarboxylase, 174
  development, 177
  in catecholamine synthesis, 182, 184
ASC transport system, 42
Ascites cells, transport of amino acids in,
    41
Ascorbate, effect on collagen synthesis, 162
  effect on tryptophan catabolism, 102
  effect on tyrosinase, 181
Asparaginase, effect on tumors, 149
  in asparagine pathway, 149
Asparagine,
  concentration in plasma, constancy, 151
  effect on asparagine pathway, 149
  pathway, 149
    development, 151
  synthetase, 149
Aspartate, N-acetylaspartate pathway, 149
  asparagine pathway, 149
  catabolic pathways, 80
  effect on creatine synthesis, 154
  in portal blood, 22
  pyrimidine pathway, 152
  transaminase, development, 63
    regulation, 62
    role in general deamination, 58
  transcarbamylase, 152
Aspartate "shuttle," 57

Atherosclerosis, effect on isovalthine excretion, 139
ATP. See *Adenosine triphosphate.*

Benzoate, effect on tyrosine catabolism, 112
Betaine, in one-carbon fragment metabolism, 165
Betaine-homocysteine transmethylase, development, 167
in one-carbon fragment metabolism, 166
Betaine transport group, 38
Bile acids, effect on isovalthine excretion, 139
Blood-brain barrier, 41
Bottle-neck effect, 6
Brain, transport of amino acids in, 41
Branched-chain amino acids, catabolic pathways, 95
circadian rhythm, 97
development, 96, 97
degradation in muscle, 24–25
effect on ornithine transaminase, 83, 84
extrahepatic degradation, 23
Branched-chain ketoaciduria, 95
Braunstein, transdeamination, 58
Bromural, effect on isovalthine excretion, 139

Calcium, effect on branched-chain amino acid catabolism, 97
effect on catecholamine storage, 186
Caloric deprivation, as catabolic-hepatotropic factor, 30
Caloric intake, as anabolic-myotropic factor, 29
Cancer, effect on alanine metabolism, 66
Carbamyl phosphate, effect on glutamate dehydrogenase, 61
effect on glutamine synthesis in liver, 130
synthetase in ornithine cycle, 121
synthetase in pyrimidine pathway, 152
Carbohydrate metabolism, regulation, 54–55
Carnitine metabolism, 172
Carnosine, in muscle, 26
synthesis in liver, 22, 24
Castration, effect on S-adenosylmethionine decarboxylase, 171
effect on ornithine decarboxylase, 171
Catabolic pathways, regulation, 16
Catabolite repression, 9
Catalase, effect on tryptophan catabolism, 102
Catechol O-methyltransferase, in catecholamine catabolism, 185

Catecholamine(s), 182
as protein-catabolic factors, 30
effect on arylamino acid decarboxylase, 176
effect on histamine synthesis, 157
effect on ornithine decarboxylase, 170
effect on phenylalanine metabolism, 109
functions, 186–187
mechanism of action, 14
metabolism, circadian rhythms, 186
development, 186
O-methyltransferase, 184
storage, 185–186
Cathepsins, in enzyme degradation, 11
Cationic transport group, 38
Cell cycle, tyrosine transaminase inducibility, 116
Cell density, effect on collagen synthesis, 161
effect on ornithine decarboxylase, 171
Cell number, in regulation, 9
Chloride, effect on aminobutyrate pathway, 147
effect on glutaminase, 132
Cholecystokinin, effect on histamine synthesis, 157
Choline, effect on carnitine metabolism, 172–173
effect on choline oxidase, 166
effect on methylation of ethanolamines, 166
in one-carbon fragment metabolism, 165
Choline oxidase, development, 167
in one-carbon fragment metabolism, 166
Chronic controls, 2
Circadian rhythms, 15
Citrate, effect on glutamine synthesis in liver, 130
excretion in alkalosis, 128
Citrulline, effect on creatine synthesis, 154
Coarse adjustments, in regulation, 2
Cobamide coenzyme, in one-carbon fragment metabolism, 165
Code, genetic, 2–3
Codon, 3
Cold, effect on alanine metabolism, 65
effect on aminobutyrate pathway, 147
effect on arylamino acid decarboxylase, 176, 184
effect on aspartate transaminase, 63
effect on carnitine metabolism, 173
effect on dopamine beta-hydroxylase, 185
effect on phenylethanolamine N-methyltransferase, 185
effect on serine catabolism, 74
effect on tryptophan catabolism, 101
effect on tyrosine hydroxylase, 184
Collagen pathway, 159
synthesis, development, 163

Collagenase, 161
Committed step, 16
Competence, 15
Complementary bases, in DNA, 3
Concentration of enzyme, in regulation, 2
Contact-inhibition, effect on tyrosine
  catabolism, 113
Cooperative effect, 7
Coordinate induction and repression,
  8–9
Co-repressor, 8
Creatine, effect on creatine synthesis, 154
  in muscle, 26
  synthesis, 153
    development, 155
    in liver, 22, 24
  transport in muscle, 41
Creatinine, excretion, 26
Cyclic adenosine monophosphate, effect on
  electrical potential of liver cell
  membrane, 46–47
  effect on glycine formation from glyoxy-
    late, 78
  effect on heme synthesis, 143
  effect on histidine catabolism, 85, 87, 88
  effect on hydroxyindole O-methyltrans-
    ferase, 176
  effect on ornithine transaminase, 83
  effect on phenylalanine metabolism, 109
  effect on serine catabolism, 74
  effect on serotonin N-acetyltransferase,
    176
  effect on thyroid hormone synthesis, 179
  effect on transport, 46
  effect on tryptophan hydroxylase, 176
  effect on tyrosine catabolism, 112, 115–
    116
  role in regulation, 12
Cyclic AMP. See *Cyclic adenosine monophosphate.*
Cycloheximide, in regulatory investigations,
  10
  site of action, 10
Cycloleucine, as model amino acid for
  transport, 38
Cycloserine, effect on aminobutyrate pathway, 148
Cysteine, catabolic pathways, 67–70
  effect on isovalthine excretion, 179
  effect on serine catabolism, 75
  effect on serine synthesis, 73
  glutathione pathways, 137–140
  taurine pathway, 137
Cysteine sulfinate decarboxylase, 137
Cystine, effect on cysteine catabolism, 70
  effect on methionine activation, 166
  effect on methionine catabolism, 92
Cystinuria, intestinal defects, 39
  kidney defects, 40
Cytidine triphosphate, effect on glutamine
  synthesis in liver, 130

Darkness, effect on hydroxyindole O-
  methyltransferase, 176
Deamination, amino acids in liver, 22
  general pathways, 58
Degradation, in regulation, 10
Deoxyribonucleic acid, in protein synthesis,
  2
Development, effect on transport of amino
  acids, 49
Developmental regulation, 15
Diabetes, effect on acetylaspartate excretion, 149
  effect on alanine metabolism, 65
  effect on aspartate transaminase, 63
  effect on betaine-homocysteine trans-
    methylase, 166
  effect on branched-chain amino acid
    catabolism, 96
  effect on carbohydrate metabolism, 54–
    55
  effect on carnitine metabolism, 173
  effect on collagen synthesis, 162
  effect on fat metabolism, 55
  effect on glutathione reductase, 139
  effect on glycine formation from
    glyoxylate, 78
  effect on glycine-serine interconversion,
    79
  effect on histidine catabolism, 85, 87
  effect on isovalthine excretion, 139
  effect on methionine activation, 165, 166
  effect on methionine catabolism, 92
  effect on ornithine cycle, 124, 126
  effect on ornithine transaminase, 83
  effect on serine catabolism, 74
  effect on serine synthesis, 73
  effect on threonine catabolism, 93
  effect on tryptophan catabolism, 101
  effect on tyrosine catabolism, 112
  muscle ribosomes in, 10
Diamine oxidase, in histamine catabolism,
  158
  in polyamine catabolism, 170
Diamino acid transport group, 38
Diaphragm, effect of insulin on amino acid
  transport, 49
Dicarbethoxydihydrocollidine, 142
Dicarboxylic acid by-pass, 57
Differentiation, 15
Diffusion, exchange, 35
  facilitated, 34
  mediated, 34
  passive, 33
Diiodotyrosine, 179
Dimethylglycine, effect on betaine-
  homocysteine transmethylase, 166
  in one-carbon fragment metabolism,
    165
Diurnal rhythms, 15
DOPA, effect on arylamino acid decarboxy-
  lase, 176, 185

DOPA (*Continued*)
  effect on tyrosine hydroxylase, 184
  in melanin synthesis, 181
Dopamine, effect on tyrosine hydroxylase, 184
  role, 182
Dopamine beta-hydroxylase, 182, 185

Effectors, 1
Efflux systems, in amino acid transport, 38
Ehrlich ascites cells, transport of amino acids in, 41
Embryo, aspartate transcarbamylase in, 152
Embryonic inducers, 15
Endocrines, in regulation, 13
End-product inhibition, 7, 16
End-product repression, 16
Epidermal growth factor, effect on ornithine decarboxylase, 170
Epinephrine, effect on arylamino acid decarboxylase, 185
  effect on carbohydrate metabolism, 54–55
  effect on fat metabolism, 55
  effect on glycine catabolism, 77
  effect on histamine synthesis, 157
  effect on isovalthine excretion, 139
  effect on phenylalanine metabolism, 109
  effect on phenylethanolamine N-methyl-transferase, 185
  effect on serine catabolism, 74
  effect on transport of amino acids, 47
  effect on tyrosine catabolism, 112, 113, 115
  role, 182
Ergoneogenesis, definition, 53
Erythrocytes, transport of amino acids in, 41
Erythropoietin, effect on heme synthesis, 143
Essential amino acids, degradation in liver, 23
Estrogen(s), effect on S-adenosylmethionine decarboxylase, 171
  effect on aminobutyrate pathway, 147–148
  effect on asparagine pathway, 149–151
  effect on aspartate transaminase, 63
  effect on aspartate transcarbamylase, 152
  effect on catechol O-methyltransferase, 185
  effect on collagen synthesis, 161
  effect on creatine synthesis, 154, 155
  effect on cysteine catabolism, 70
  effect on glycine-serine interconversion, 79
  effect on histamine catabolism, 158
  effect on histamine synthesis, 157
  effect on histidine catabolism, 87
  effect on melanin synthesis, 181
  effect on methionine activation, 165

Estrogen(s) (*Continued*)
  effect on methionine catabolism, 92
  effect on methyl group synthesis, 167
  effect on ornithine decarboxylase, 170
  effect on ornithine transaminase, 83, 84
  effect on serotonin N-acetyltransferase, 176
  effect on taurine pathway, 137
  effect on transport of amino acids, 47
  effect on tryptophan catabolism, 101
Ethanolamine(s), in one-carbon fragment metabolism, 165
  transmethylase, development, 167
Eukaryotes, regulation in, 4
Exchange diffusion, 35

Facilitated diffusion, 34
Families of amino acids, 64–65
Fasting, effect on alanine metabolism, 65
  effect on aspartate transaminase, 63
  effect on betaine-homocysteine trans-methylase, 166
  effect on branched-chain amino acid catabolism, 96, 97
  effect on carbohydrate metabolism, 54–55
  effect on carnitine metabolism, 173
  effect on cysteine catabolism, 70
  effect on fat metabolism, 55
  effect on glutamate dehydrogenase, 61
  effect on glutamine synthesis in liver, 130
  effect on glycine formation from glyoxyl-ate, 78
  effect on glycine-serine interconversion, 79
  effect on heme synthesis, 143
  effect on histamine synthesis, 157
  effect on histidine catabolism, 85, 87, 88
  effect on methionine activation, 165
  effect on methionine catabolism, 92
  effect on methyl group synthesis, 167
  effect on ornithine cycle, 124
  effect on ornithine transaminase, 83, 84
  effect on phenylalanine metabolism, 109
  effect on proline catabolism, 90
  effect on sarcosine dehydrogenase, 166
  effect on serine catabolism, 74
  effect on serine synthesis, 73
  effect on threonine catabolism, 93
  effect on tryptophan catabolism, 101, 102
  effect on tyrosine catabolism, 112
Fat, effect on carnitine metabolism, 173
  effect on choline oxidase, 166
  metabolism, regulation, 55
Feedback, 7
Fine adjustments, in regulation, 2
Fluoroacetate, effect on acetylaspartate accumulation in brain, 149
Folate, effect on glycine-serine intercon-version, 79

Folate (*Continued*)
  effect on histidine catabolism, 88
Follicle-stimulating hormone, effect on
    ornithine decarboxylase, 170
  effect on transport of amino acids, 48
Formyl-tetrahydrofolate, effect on glycine-
    serine interconversion, 79
  effect on threonine catabolism, 93

Gastrin, effect on histamine synthesis, 157
Gastrointestinal tract, role in amino acid
    metabolism, 20
Gene, types, 8
Glucagon, as catabolic-hepatotropic factor,
    30
  effect on alanine metabolism, 65
  effect on aspartate transaminase, 63
  effect on carbohydrate metabolism, 54–55
  effect on cysteine catabolism, 70
  effect on fat metabolism, 55
  effect on glycine formation from glyoxy-
    late, 78
  effect on heme synthesis, 143
  effect on histidine catabolism, 85, 87, 88
  effect on lysine catabolism, 99
  effect on methionine catabolism, 92
  effect on ornithine cycle, 124
  effect on ornithine decarboxylase, 170
  effect on ornithine transaminase, 83
  effect on phenylalanine metabolism, 109
  effect on phenylethanolamine N-methyl-
    transferase, 185
  effect on serine catabolism, 74
  effect on serine synthesis, 73
  effect on transport of amino acids, 47
  effect on tryptophan catabolism, 102
  effect on tyrosine catabolism, 112, 113,
    115–116
  mechanism of action, 14
Glucocorticoids, as catabolic-hepatotropic
    factors, 30
  effect on alanine metabolism, 65
  effect on aminobutyrate pathway, 147
  effect on asparagine pathway, 151
  effect on aspartate transaminase, 63
  effect on betaine-homocysteine trans-
    methylase, 166
  effect on branched-chain amino acid
    catabolism, 96
  effect on carbohydrate metabolism, 54–
    55
  effect on collagen catabolism, 162
  effect on collagen synthesis, 162
  effect on cysteine catabolism, 70
  effect on fat metabolism, 55
  effect on glutamate dehydrogenase, 61
  effect on glutamine synthesis in liver, 130
  effect on glycine catabolism, 77
  effect on glycine-glucose conversion, 77

Glucocorticoids (*Continued*)
  effect on glycine-serine interconversion,
    79
  effect on heme synthesis, 143
  effect on histamine synthesis, 157
  effect on histidine catabolism, 85, 87, 88
  effect on isovalthine excretion, 179
  effect on lysine catabolism, 99
  effect on lysosomal membranes, 11
  effect on melanin synthesis, 181
  effect on methionine activation, 165
  effect on methionine catabolism, 92
  effect on methyl group synthesis, 167
  effect on ornithine cycle, 124
  effect on ornithine decarboxylase, 170
  effect on ornithine transaminase, 83
  effect on phenylalanine metabolism, 109
  effect on phenylethanolamine N-methyl-
    transferase, 185
  effect on proline catabolism, 90
  effect on serine catabolism, 74
  effect on serine synthesis, 73
  effect on taurine pathway, 137
  effect on threonine catabolism, 93
  effect on transport of amino acids, 46
  effect on tryptophan catabolism, 102, 104,
    105
  effect on tryptophan hydroxylase, 176
  effect on tyrosine catabolism, 112, 113,
    115, 116
Glucogenic amino acids, definition, 52
  pathways of disposal of carbon, 57
Gluconeogenesis, definition, 52
  factors favoring, 30
  from amino acids, 52–53
  in liver, 22, 24
  in acidosis, 133
Glucosamine, effect on tyrosine catabolism,
    112
Glucose, effect on alanine metabolism, 66
  effect on aspartate transaminase, 63
  effect on cysteine catabolism, 70
  effect on glutamate dehydrogenase, 61
  effect on glycine-glucose conversion, 77
  effect on glycine-serine interconversion,
    79
  effect on heme synthesis, 143
  effect on histidine catabolism, 87, 88
  effect on methionine metabolism, 92
  effect on ornithine cycle, 126
  effect on ornithine transaminase, 83, 84
  effect on serine catabolism, 75
  effect on tryptophan catabolism, 102
  effect on tyrosine catabolism, 113
Glucose effect, 9
Glutamate, catabolic pathways, 80
  effect on aminobutyrate pathway, 147
  effect on glutaminase in brain, 146
  effect on glutaminase in kidney, 132, 133
  effect on ornithine transaminase, 84
  effect on tyrosine catabolism, 112

Glutamate (*Continued*)
  glutamine pathway in nervous tissue, 145
  in portal blood, 22
Glutamate decarboxylase, 147
Glutamate dehydrogenase, development, 62
  regulation of, 60
  role in deamination, 58, 62
  role in reamination, 62
  role in synthesis of nonessential amino acids, 62
Glutamate-oxaloacetate transaminase. See *Aspartate transaminase.*
Glutaminase, development, 134
  in acidosis, 131–132
  in nervous system, 146
Glutaminase I. See *Glutaminase.*
Glutaminase II. See *Glutamine-keto acid transaminase.*
Glutamine, effect on glutamine synthesis in culture, 130
  in portal blood, 22, 24
  pathway for ammonia disposal, 127
  pathway in nervous tissue, 145
  synthesis, comparative aspects, 134
    in brain and retina, development, 145–146
    in liver, 22, 24, 128, 130
      development, 130
  synthetase, in brain and retina, 145
    in kidney, 132–133, 134
Glutamine-keto acid transaminase, in acidosis, 131
γ-Glutamyl cycle, in amino acid transport, 39
Glutamylcysteine synthetase, 137
Glutathione, effect on glutathione synthesis, 137
  effect on thyroidal peroxidase, 179
  in portal blood, 22, 24
  pathways, 137–140
  role in renal amino acid transport, 39
  synthesis in liver, 22, 24
Glutathione peroxidase, 139
Glutathione reductase, 139
Glutathione synthetase, 137
Glyceraldehyde-3-phosphate, effect on aspartate transaminase, 63
Glycine, catabolic pathways, 75, 77–80
  development, 72
  effect on creatine synthesis, 154
  effect on glutamine synthesis in brain, 145
  effect on glutamine synthesis in liver, 130
  effect on glycine synthesis, 77
  formation from glyoxylate, development, 78
  heme pathway, 141
  in one-carbon fragment metabolism, 165
  porphyrin pathway, 141
  purine pathway, 140
  synthesis, 77, 79–80

Glycine oxidase, in acidosis, 131
Glycine-serine interconversion, 79
Granuloma, effect on collagen synthesis, 161
Growth, effect on collagen synthesis, 161
  effect on histidine catabolism, 87, 88
  effect on transport of amino acids, 49
Growth hormone, as anabolic-myotropic factor, 29
  deficiency, as catabolic factor, 30
  effect on S-adenosylmethionine decarboxylase, 171
  effect on alanine metabolism, 66
  effect on amino acid deposition in muscle, 29
  effect on aspartate transaminase, 63
  effect on branched-chain amino acid catabolism, 96
  effect on collagen synthesis, 161
  effect on creatine synthesis, 154, 155
  effect on fat metabolism, 55
  effect on glutamate dehydrogenase, 61
  effect on glutaminase, 132
  effect on histidine catabolism, 87
  effect on methyl group synthesis, 167
  effect on ornithine cycle, 126
  effect on ornithine decarboxylase, 170
  effect on ornithine transaminase, 83
  effect on serine catabolism, 75
  effect on serine synthesis, 73
  effect on transport of amino acids, 44
  effect on tryptophan catabolism, 102
  effect on tyrosine catabolism, 113
Growth-promoting polypeptides, effect on transport of amino acids, 44
Guanidino transport group, 38
Guanidoacetate, effect on creatine synthesis, 155
  transmethylase, 153–154

Hartnup disease, intestinal defect, 39
  kidney defect, 39
Heat, effect on histamine synthesis, 157–158
Heme, effect on globin synthesis, 144
  effect on heme synthesis, 141, 143
  effect on hemoglobin synthesis, 144
  effect on tryptophan catabolism, 101–102
  pathway, 141
  synthesis, development, 143
Hemoglobin synthesis, 144
  development, 144
Hepatotropic factors, 30
Hexose monophosphate shunt pathway in acidotic kidney, 128
Hibernation, effect on aminobutyrate pathway, 147
Histaminase. See *Diamine oxidase.*

Histamine, effect on histamine catabolism, 158
effect on histamine synthesis, 158
pathway, 155
development, 158
Histidine, catabolic pathways, 85
development, 87, 88
circadian rhythm in intestinal transport, 49
effect on glutamine synthesis in brain, 145
effect on histamine catabolism, 158
histamine pathway, 155
Histidine decarboxylase, 155
Histidinemia, 85
Histones, effect on tryptophan catabolism, 102
effect on tyrosine catabolism, 112
in eukaryotic nuclei, 4
phosphorylation of, 12
Homocysteine, effect on ornithine transaminase, 84
Homogentisate, effect on tyrosine catabolism, 113, 115
Hormones, in regulation, 13
Hydrazines, effect on aminobutyrate pathway, 148
Hydroxyindoleacetate, 174
Hydroxyindole O-methyltransferase, 174
Hydroxylamines, effect on aminobutyrate pathway, 148
Hydroxyproline. See *Proline.*
Hypercholesterolemia, effect on isovalthine excretion, 139
Hyperiminoglycinuria, 40
Hypertension, effect on collagen synthesis, 161–162
effect on histamine synthesis, 157
Hypertrophy, cardiac, effect on S-adenosylmethionine decarboxylase, 171
effect on ornithine decarboxylase, 170
renal, effect on aspartate transcarbamylase, 152
Hypocholesterolemic drugs, effect on isovalthine excretion, 139
Hypophysectomy, effect on S-adenosylmethionine decarboxylase, 171
effect on alanine metabolism, 65
effect on aspartate transaminase, 63
effect on branched-chain amino acid catabolism, 96
effect on catechol O-methyltransferase, 185
effect on dopamine beta-hydroxylase, 185
effect on glutamate dehydrogenase, 61
effect on glycine catabolism, 77
effect on histamine catabolism, 158
effect on histidine catabolism, 87
effect on monoamine oxidase, 176, 185
effect on ornithine decarboxylase, 171

Hypophysectomy (*Continued*)
effect on phenylethanolamine N-methyltransferase, 185
effect on proline catabolism, 90
effect on serine catabolism, 75
effect on tryptophan catabolism, 101
effect on tyrosine hydroxylase, 184
Hypothalamic stimulation, effect on tryptophan catabolism, 101
Hypothalamus, effect on melanin synthesis, 181
effect on thyroid hormone synthesis, 179
Hypothyroidism, effect on isovalthine excretion, 139
Hypoxia, effect on hemoglobin synthesis, 145
Hysteretic enzymes, 2

Imbalanced amino acid diet, effect on alanine metabolism, 65
effect on aspartate transaminase, 63
Iminoglycine transport group, 38
Iminoglycinuria, 40
Indoleamines, effect on tyrosine catabolism, 112
Inducer, action of, 8
embryonic, 15
Induction, coordinate, 8–9
definition, 2
mechanism, 7
Infection, effect on histamine synthesis, 157
Inhibition, by end-product, 7
by metabolite, 7
definition, 2
Inosinate, effect on purine synthesis, 141
Insulin, as anabolic-myotropic factor, 29
deficiency, as catabolic factor, 30
effect on amino acid deposition in muscle, 29
effect on aminobutyrate pathway, 147
effect on carbohydrate metabolism, 54–55
effect on collagen synthesis, 161, 162
effect on fat metabolism, 55
effect on glutathione reductase, 139
effect on glycine-glucose conversion, 77
effect on glycine-serine interconversion, 79
effect on histamine synthesis, 157
effect on isovalthine excretion, 139
effect on ornithine cycle, 126
effect on ornithine decarboxylase, 170
effect on phenylethanolamine N-methyltransferase, 185
effect on serine catabolism, 75
effect on serine synthesis, 73
effect on threonine catabolism, 93

Insulin (*Continued*)
  effect on transport of amino acids, 44, 49
    development, 49
  effect on tryptophan catabolism, 102
  effect on tyrosine catabolism, 112, 113, 115
  secretion stimulated by amino acids, 29
  secretion stimulated by glucose, 29
Intestinal bacteria, role in nitrogen metabolism, 22
Intestinal flora. See *Intestinal bacteria*.
Intestine, transport of amino acids in, 38
  during development, 49
Irreversible reactions, regulation, 16
Isoenzymes in regulation, 13
Isolation, effect on phenylethanolamine N-methyltransferase, 185
  effect on tyrosine hydroxylase, 184
Isoleucine. See *Branched-chain amino acids*.
Isovalerate, conjugation with glutathione, 139
  effect on isovalthine excretion, 139
Isovaleric acidemia, 140
N-Isovalerylglycine, 140
Isovalthine pathway, 139
Isozymes. See *Isoenzymes*.

Keratinocytes, 181
Ketogenic amino acids, definition, 52
  pathways of disposal of carbon, 56
Ketoglutarate, effect on glutamine synthesis in liver, 130
  excretion in alkalosis, 128
Ketone bodies, effect on methionine activation, 166
Kidney, acidification of urine, 128
  role in amino acid metabolism, 26
  role in gluconeogenesis, 60
  transport of amino acids in, 39
    during development, 49
Krebs cycle, effect of ATP, 55
Kwashiorkor, 31

"L" transport system, 37
Lac operon, 8
Lactate, effect on collagen synthesis, 162
Late fetal stage, in development, 15
Late suckling stage, in development, 15
Leucine. See also *Branched-chain amino acids*.
  effect on branched-chain amino acid catabolism, 96
  effect on isovalthine excretion, 139
  effect on ornithine cycle, 126
  effect on tyrosine catabolism, 112
"Leucine-preferring" transport system, 37
Leukocytes, transport of amino acids in, 41

Light, effect on arylamino acid decarboxylase, 176, 184
  effect on hydroxyindole O-methyltransferase, 176
  effect on serotonin N-acetyltransferase, 176
Lipoproteins, in portal blood, 22
Liver, fibrosis, effect on collagen synthesis, 161
  role in amino acid metabolism, 22
  transport of amino acids in, 40
    during development, 49
Long-term controls, 2
Luteinizing hormone, effect on ornithine decarboxylase, 170
Lysine, carnitine pathway, 172
  catabolic pathways, 98
  collagen pathway, 159
  effect on arginase, 82
  effect on ornithine cycle, 126
Lysolecithin, effect on phenylalanine metabolism, 109
Lysosomes, in enzyme degradation, 11

Magnesium, effect on catecholamine storage, 186
Malate "shuttle," 57
Maleate, effect on glutaminase, 131–132
Manganese, effect on ornithine cycle, 126
Maple syrup urine disease, 95
Marasmus, 31
Mass action, in regulation, 1, 6
Mediated diffusion, 34
Melanin pathway, 181
Melanocytes, 181
Melanocyte-stimulating hormones, effect on melanin synthesis, 181
Melanosomes, 181
Melatonin, circadian rhythm, 177
  development, 178
  effect on melanin synthesis, 181
  metabolism, 174
Membrane transport, in regulation, 6
Mercaptopurine, effect on purine synthesis, 141
Mercapturic acids, 139
Messenger ribonucleic acid, in protein synthesis, 3
Metabolite inhibition, 7
"Methiamine," 170
Methionine, activating enzyme, development, 167
  activation, 163
  catabolic pathways, 90
    development, 92
  effect on alanine metabolism, 65
  effect on aspartate transaminase, 63

Methionine (*Continued*)
  effect on betaine-homocysteine trans-
    methylase, 166
  effect on choline oxidase, 166
  effect on cysteine catabolism, 70
  effect on isovalthine excretion, 139
  effect on methionine activation, 166
  effect on methionine catabolism, 92
  effect on methyl group synthesis, 167
  effect on ornithine transaminase, 84
  effect on serine synthesis, 73
  effect on taurine pathway, 137
  effect on tyrosine catabolism, 112
  methyl group pathways, 163
Methionine sulfoximine synthesis in brain,
    145
Methyl-donors, effect on betaine-homo-
    cysteine transmethylase, 166
  effect on choline oxidase, 166
Methyl group, effect of vitamin B$_{12}$ on
    synthesis, 167
  pathways, 163
  synthesis, 167
    development, 167
3-Methylhistidine, in muscle, 26
Methyl-tetrahydrofolate, effect on
    glycine-serine interconversion, 79
  effect on threonine catabolism, 93
Mitotic rate, effect on aspartate transcar-
    bamylase, 152
Modulators, 1, 6–7
Monoamine oxidase, development, 177
  in catecholamine catabolism, 184, 185
  in histamine pathway, 158
  in indoleamine catabolism, 174
Monoiodotyrosine, 179
Mucopolysaccharides, effect on tyrosine
    hydroxylase, 184
Mucosal cells, metabolic activities, 20–22
Multi-enzyme particles, in regulation, 6
Muscle, necrosis, effect on taurine path-
    way, 137
  role in amino acid metabolism, 24
  transport of amino acids in, 41
Myotropic factors, 29
Myxedema, effect on isovalthine excre-
    tion, 139

Negative feedback, 7
Negative nitrogen balance, factors favoring,
    30
Neonatal stage in development, 15
Nephrosis, effect on isovalthine excretion,
    139
Nerves, in regulation, 14
Neural regulation, 14
Neuraminate, effect on glutamine syn-
    thesis in brain, 145

Neurohormones, in regulation, 14
Neutral transport groups, 37
Nicotinamide, effect on choline oxidase, 166
  effect on tryptophan catabolism, 102
  sparing of requirement by tryptophan,
    101
Nicotinamide adenine dinucleotide, effect
    on glutamine synthesis in liver, 130
  effect on glutathione synthesis, 137
Nicotinamide adenine dinucleotide phos-
    phate, effect on glutathione peroxi-
    dase, 139
  effect on tryptophan catabolism, 102
  in acidosis, 133
NIH shift, 108–109
Nitrogen balance, definition, 29
  negative, factors favoring, 30
  positive, factors favoring, 29
Nonessential amino acids, degradation in
    muscle, 24
  synthesis in liver, 22
Norepinephrine, effect on arylamino acid
    decarboxylase, 185
  effect on hydroxyindole O-methyltrans-
    ferase, 176
  effect on phenylethanolamine N-methyl-
    transferase, 185
  effect on serotonin N-acetyltransferase,
    176
  effect on tryptophan hydroxylase, 176
  effect on tyrosine hydroxylase, 184
  role, 182
Nucleic acids, in protein synthesis, 2
Nucleoside phosphates, effect on purine
    synthesis, 141
Nucleotides, effect on glutamate dehydro-
    genase, 61
  effect on glutamine synthesis in brain,
    145
  effect on purine synthesis, 141
  effect on serine catabolism, 74
  effect on tyrosine catabolism, 112

Obesity, starvation therapy in, 31
One-carbon unit metabolism, 163–168
  effect of S-adenosylhomocysteine, 166
  effect of S-adenosylmethionine, 166
Operator, 8
Operon, 8
Ornithine, effect on arginase, 82
  effect on ornithine cycle, 126
  effect on ornithine transaminase, 84
Ornithine cycle, 121
  bioenergetics, 123
  developmental regulation, 127
  intracellular localization, 123
  specific activities of enzymes, 123
Ornithine decarboxylase, 168, 170

Ornithine transaminase, development, 84
  regulation, 83
  role in metabolism, 84–85, 124
Ornithine transcarbamylase, 121
Ouabain, inhibitor of amino acid transport, 39
Ovariectomy, effect on tryptophan catabolism, 102
"Overshoot," in development of tryptophan pyrrolase, 106
Oxygen, effect on aminobutyrate pathway, 147
  effect on tyrosine hydroxylase, 184

Parasympathetic stimulation, effect on histamine synthesis, 157
  effect on hydroxyindole O-methyltransferase, 176
Parathyroid hormone, effect on collagen synthesis, 161
  effect on transport of amino acids, 48
Passive diffusion, 33
Pentose shunt pathway in acidotic kidney, 128
Permease, 35
Peroxide, effect on tryptophan catabolism, 102
Phenolic acids, effect on aminobutyrate pathway, 147–148
Phenylalanine, effect on phenylalanine metabolism, 109
  effect on tyrosinase, 181
  metabolic pathways, 107
    circadian rhythm, 109
    development, 109
Phenylethanolamine N-methyltransferase, 182, 185
Phosphate, effect on aminobutyrate pathway, 147
  effect on branched-chain amino acid catabolism, 97
  effect on glutaminase in brain, 146
  effect on glutaminase in kidney, 131–132
  effect on glutamine synthesis in liver, 130
Phosphocreatine, in muscle, 26
Phosphohydroxypyruvate, effect on serine catabolism, 74
Phosphoribosyl pyrophosphate, amidotransferase, 141
  effect on pyrimidine synthesis, 152
Phosphorylation, in activation of enzymes, 12
Phytohemagglutinin, effect on ornithine decarboxylase, 170
  effect on pyrimidine synthesis, 152
Pituitary factor, effect on histidine catabolism, 87

Pituitary lipolytic fraction, effect on serine catabolism, 74
Placenta, transport of amino acids in, 49
Plasma proteins, degradation, in liver, 24
  in muscle, 24
  synthesis in liver, 22
Polyamine(s), biological role, 172
  catabolism, 170
  metabolic pathways, 168
  synthesis, circadian rhythm, 171–172
    development, 171
Polyribosome, in protein synthesis, 3
Polysome. See *Polyribosome.*
Porphyria, 142
Porphyrin pathway, 141
Positive nitrogen balance, factors favoring, 29
Pregnancy, effect on alanine metabolism, 66
  effect on carnitine metabolism, 173
  effect on tryptophan catabolism, 101
Pregnanolone, effect on heme synthesis, 143
Procollagen, 159
Procollagenase, 161
Progesterone, effect on cysteine catabolism, 70
  effect on methionine catabolism, 92
Prokaryotes, regulation in, 3
Proline, catabolic pathways, 88
  collagen pathway, 159
  effect on arginase, 82
  effect on ornithine cycle, 126
  effect on ornithine transaminase, 84
  effect on proline catabolism, 90
  effect on proline synthesis, 90
  effect on tyrosine catabolism, 112
  synthesis, 88
Propylamine transferases, 170
Prostaglandins, effect on catecholamine storage, 186
Protamines in eukaryotic nuclei, 4
Protein, as anabolic-myotropic factor, 29
  catabolism, factors favoring, 29
  effect on alanine metabolism, 65
  effect on aminobutyrate pathway, 147
  effect on asparagine pathway, 151
  effect on aspartate transaminase, 63
  effect on betaine-homocysteine transmethylase, 166
  effect on branched-chain amino acid catabolism, 95–96, 97
  effect on choline oxidase, 166
  effect on creatine synthesis, 154
  effect on cysteine catabolism, 70
  effect on glutamate dehydrogenase, 61
  effect on glutaminase, 132
  effect on glutamine synthesis in liver, 130
  effect on glycine catabolism, 77
  effect on glycine-serine interconversion, 79
  effect on histidine catabolism, 85, 87, 88

Protein (*Continued*)
  effect on lysine catabolism, 99
  effect on methionine activation, 165
  effect on methionine catabolism, 92
  effect on methyl group synthesis, 167
  effect on ornithine cycle, 124
  effect on ornithine transaminase, 83
  effect on phenylalanine metabolism,
    109
  effect on proline catabolism, 90
  effect on serine catabolism, 74, 75
  effect on serine synthesis, 73
  effect on taurine pathway, 137
  effect on transport of amino acids, 48
  effect on tryptophan catabolism, 101
  effect on tyrosine catabolism, 112, 113,
    115
  plasma, degradation, in liver, 24
    in muscle, 24
    synthesis, in liver, 22
  synthesis, factors favoring, 29
  turnover, in gastrointestinal tract, 20
    rate in various tissues, 30
Protein-caloric deprivation, 31
Protein deprivation, as catabolic-hepato-
    tropic factor, 30
Protein-sparing effects, 29
Protocollagen, 159
Protyrosinase, 181
Purine nucleotides, effect on purine syn-
    thesis, 141
Purine synthesis, 140
Puromycin, effect on tryptophan pyrrolase
    induction, 102
  in regulatory investigations, 10
  site of action, 10
Putreanine, 170
Putrescine, effect on S-adenosylmethionine
    decarboxylase, 171
  effect on ornithine decarboxylase, 171
  effect on spermine synthase, 171
  metabolism, 168
Pyridoxine, effect on aminobutyrate path-
    way, 148
  effect on arylamino acid decarboxylase,
    176, 184–185
  effect on cysteine catabolism, 70
  effect on histamine synthesis, 155, 157
  effect on histidine catabolism, 87
  effect on methionine catabolism, 92
  effect on taurine pathway, 137
  effect on transport of amino acids, 48
  effect on tyrosine catabolism, 112, 113
  interrelation with thyroid hormones, 70–
    71
Pyrimidines, synthesis, 152
  development, 152–153
Pyruvate, effect on phenylalanine metabo-
    lism, 109
Pyruvoneogenesis, 53

Quinolinate, effect on gluconeogenesis,
    99, 101
  effect on tyrosine catabolism, 112

Rate-limiting reactions, regulation, 16
Redundancy, regulatory, 17
Regeneration, effect on S-adenosyl-
    methionine decarboxylase, 171
  effect on alanine metabolism, 66
  effect on asparagine pathway, 149
  effect on aspartate transcarbamylase, 152
  effect on branched-chain amino acid
    catabolism, 96
  effect on glutamine synthesis in liver, 130
  effect on lysine catabolism, 99
  effect on ornithine decarboxylase, 170
  effect on ornithine transaminase, 83
Regulation, types, 1–2
Regulator gene, 8
Regulatory redundancy, 17
Renotropic effects, 45
Replication, 3
Repression, catabolite, 9
  coordinate, 8–9
  definition, 2
  mechanism, 7
Repressor, action, 8
  in tyrosine transaminase regulation, 115
Reticulocytes, transport of amino acids in,
    41
Rhythmic regulation, 15
Riboflavin, effect on choline oxidase, 166
Ribosomes, in protein synthesis, 3
  in regulation, 10

Salicylates, effect on aminobutyrate path-
    way, 147–148
Sarcosine, in one-carbon fragment
    metabolism, 165
Sarcosine dehydrogenase, 166
  development, 167
Scurvy, effect on collagen synthesis, 162
Seasons, tyrosine transaminase variation,
    116
Second messenger. See *Cyclic adenosine
    monophosphate.*
Secretion, regulation of, 11
Senescence, tyrosine transaminase induci-
    bility, 116
Serine, catabolic pathways, 74
  development, 75
  effect on glutamine synthesis in liver, 130
  effect on serine synthesis, 73
  in one-carbon fragment metabolism, 165
  synthetic pathways, 71–73
  development, 73

Serotonin, N-acetyltransferase, 174
  circadian rhythm, 177
  effect on arylamino acid decarboxylase, 176, 185
  effect on serotonin synthesis, 176
  metabolism, 174
  development, 177
Short-term controls, 2
Shuttle mechanisms, 57
Sialate, effect on glutamine synthesis of brain, 145
Size of mammal, relation to serine catabolism, 74–75
Sodium, effect on catecholamine storage, 186
  role in amino acid transport, 38–39
Sodium-potassium activated ATPases, 39
Somatotropic hormone. See *Growth hormone.*
Specific activity, in regulation, 1
Spermidine, effect on ornithine decarboxylase, 171
  metabolism, 168
Spermine, effect on ornithine decarboxylase, 171
  metabolism, 168
Spermine synthase, 171
Starvation, decreased amino acid catabolism in, 31
  effect on asparagine pathway, 151
  metabolism in, 31
Steroid hormones, effect on glutamate dehydrogenase, 61
  effect on heme synthesis, 143
  mechanism of action, 14
Stimulation (neural), effect on catecholamine storage, 186
Storage granules, in secretion, 11
Stress, as catabolic-hepatotropic factor, 30
  effect on dopamine beta-hydroxylase, 185
  effect on histamine synthesis in skin, 157
  effect on ornithine decarboxylase, 170
  effect on phenylethanolamine N-methyltransferase, 185
  effect on tryptophan hydroxylase, 176
  effect on tyrosine hydroxylase, 184
Structural gene, 8
Sugars, effect on transport of amino acids, 38, 50
Sulfur deficiency, effect on methyl group synthesis, 167
"Superinduction," by actinomycin, 105
  of tyrosine transaminase, 113
Sympathetic stimulation, effect on dopamine beta-hydroxylase, 185
  effect on hydroxyindole O-methyltransferase, 176
  effect on phenylethanolamine N-methyltransferase, 185

Sympathetic stimulation (*Continued*)
  effect on serotonin N-acetyltransferase, 176
  effect on tyrosine hydroxylase, 184

Taurine, in muscle, 26
  pathway, 137
  synthesis in liver, 22, 24
Testosterone, as anabolic-myotropic factor, 29
  deficiency, as catabolic factor, 30
  effect on S-adenosylmethionine decarboxylase, 171
  effect on amino acid deposition in muscle, 29
  effect on arginase, 82
  effect on asparagine pathway, 149–151
  effect on collagen synthesis, 161
  effect on creatine synthesis, 154
  effect on glycine catabolism, 77
  effect on glycine-serine interconversion, 79
  effect on histamine catabolism, 158
  effect on methionine activation, 165
  effect on methionine catabolism, 92
  effect on ornithine decarboxylase, 170
  effect on transport of amino acids, 45, 47
  effect on tryptophan catabolism, 102
  renotropic effects of, 45
Tetrahydrofolate, effect on methyl group synthesis, 167
  in one-carbon fragment metabolism, 165
Thiamine, effect on choline oxidase, 166
  effect on histidine catabolism, 87, 88
Thiosemicarbazide, effect on aminobutyrate pathway, 148
Threonine, catabolic pathways, 93
  effect on creatine synthesis, 154
Thyroglobulin, 179
Thyroidectomy, effect on cysteine catabolism, 70
  effect on glycine catabolism, 77
  effect on tyrosine hydroxylase, 184
Thyroid hormones, as catabolic-hepatotropic factors, 30
  development, 179
  effect on arylamino acid decarboxylase, 176, 184
  effect on aspartate transaminase, 63
  effect on betaine-homocysteine transmethylase, 166
  effect on catechol O-methyltransferase, 185
  effect on choline oxidase, 166
  effect on collagen catabolism, 162
  effect on collagen synthesis, 161
  effect on creatine synthesis, 154, 155
  effect on cysteine catabolism, 70

Thyroid hormones (*Continued*)
  effect on fat metabolism, 55
  effect on glutamate dehydrogenase, 61
  effect on glutamine synthesis, in liver, 130
    in retina, 145
  effect on glycine catabolism, 77
  effect on heme synthesis, 143
  effect on histamine catabolism, 158
  effect on histidine catabolism, 85, 87, 88
  effect on melanin synthesis, 181
  effect on methionine activation, 165
  effect on methionine catabolism, 92
  effect on monoamine oxidase, 176, 185
  effect on ornithine cycle, 124
  effect on ornithine decarboxylase, 170
  effect on proline catabolism, 90
  effect on serine catabolism, 75
  effect on taurine pathway, 137
  effect on thyroid hormone synthesis, 179
  effect on transport of amino acids, 45
  effect on tryptophan catabolism, 105–106
  effect on tyrosine catabolism, 112, 113, 115
  in growth and differentiation, 29
  interrelation with pyridoxine, 70–71
  synthesis, 179
Thyrotropic hormone, effect on fat metabolism, 55
  effect on thyroid hormone synthesis, 179
  effect on transport of amino acids, 48
Thyroxine. See also *Thyroid hormones.*
  pathway, 179
Tourniquet injury, effect on tyrosine catabolism, 115
Tourniquet shock, effect on histamine synthesis, 157
Transamidinase, half-life, 155
  in creatine pathway, 153–154
Transaminases. See under individual enzymes.
Transamination, role in general deamination, 58
Transcription, 3
Transdeamination, definition, 58
Transfer ribonucleic acid, in protein synthesis, 3
  in regulation, 9–10
Translation, 3
Translocation, amino acids, 27–29
Transport, active, 35
  amino acid groups, 36
  as mechanism of regulation, 6
  circadian rhythm in, 49
  effect of adrenocorticotropic hormone, 48
  effect of cyclic adenosine monophosphate, 46
  effect of dietary protein, 48
  effect of epinephrine, 47
  effect of estrogens, 47
  effect of follicle-stimulating hormone, 48

Transport (*Continued*)
  effect of glucagon, 47
  effect of glucocorticoids, 46
  effect of growth hormone, 44
  effect of growth-promoting polypeptides, 44
  effect of insulin, 44
  effect of insulin during development, 49
  effect of parathyroid hormone, 48
  effect of pyridoxine deficiency, 48
  effect of sugars, 38, 50
  effect of testosterone, 45, 47
  effect of thyroid hormones, 45
  effect of thyrotropic hormone, 48
  effect of vitamin E deficiency, 48
  in brain, 41
  in diaphragm during development, 49
  in Ehrlich ascites cells, 41
  in erythrocytes, 41
  in intestine, 38
    during development, 49
  in kidney, 39
    during development, 49
  in leukocytes, 41
  in liver, 40
    during development, 49
  in muscle, 41
  in placenta, 49
  in reticulocytes, 41
  regulation, 42
  types, 33
Triiodothyronine, 179
Tropocollagen, 159
Tryptophan, catabolic pathways, 99
  circadian rhythm, 107
  development, 106
  deficiency in Hartnup disease, 49
  effect on gluconeogenesis, 99, 101
  effect on histamine catabolism, 158
  effect on nicotinamide requirement, 101
  effect on ornithine cycle, 126–127
  effect on phenylalanine metabolism, 109
  effect on polyribosomes, 10
  effect on tryptophan catabolism, 102, 104
  effect on tyrosine catabolism, 112, 117
  melatonin pathway, 174
  serotonin pathway, 174
Tryptophan hydroxylase, development, 177
  in indoleamine pathway, 174
Tryptophan pyrrolase. See *Tryptophan catabolic pathways.*
Tumors, effect on asparagine pathway, 149
  effect on histamine synthesis, 157
Turnover, protein, in various tissues, 30
Tyramine, effect on catecholamine storage, 186
Tyrosinase, development, 182
  in melanin pathway, 181
Tyrosine, catabolic pathways, 110
  circadian rhythm, 116, 117

Tyrosine (*Continued*)
    catabolic pathways, development, 115
    catecholamine pathway, 182
    effect on phenylalanine metabolism, 109
    effect on tyrosine catabolism, 110, 115
    melanin pathway, 181
    thyroid hormone pathway, 179
Tyrosine hydroxylase, in catecholamine
    pathway, 182, 184
Tyrosine transaminase, circadian rhythm,
    116
    half-life, 116
    isoenzymes, 112
    regulation, 110

Urate, excretion, 26
Urea, excretion, 26
    recycling, 22
    role of liver in synthesis, 24
    synthesis, 121. See also *Ornithine cycle.*
Urease, bacterial, 22
Uridine triphosphate, effect on pyrimidine
    synthesis, 152

Vagal stimulation, effect on histamine
    synthesis, 157
Valine. See also *Branched-chain amino acids.*
    effect on ornithine cycle, 126
Vanilmandelate, 184
Vitamin A, effect on collagen catabolism,
    162–163
Vitamin B6. See *Pyridoxine.*
Vitamin B12, effect on choline oxidase, 166
    effect on methyl group synthesis, 167
    in one-carbon fragment metabolism, 165
Vitamin E, effect of deficiency on trans-
    port of amino acids, 48
    effect on creatine synthesis, 154

Weaning stage in development, 15
Wound healing, effect on collagen
    synthesis, 161

Zeitgeber, 15
Zymogens, in regulation, 11